The New Holistic Way for Dogs and Cats

The Stress-Health Connection

Paul McCutcheon, DVM
and Susan Weinstein

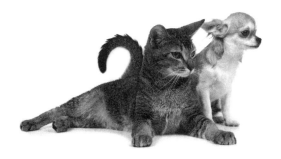

CELESTIAL ARTS
Berkeley

Copyright © 2010 by Paul McCutcheon, DVM, and Susan Weinstein

Published in the United States by Celestial Arts, an imprint of the
Crown Publishing Group, a division of Random House, Inc., New York.
www.crownpublishing.com
www.tenspeed.com

All the case studies that appear in this book are real or are composits of real cases and are used with permission. The names of certain clients and patients have been altered, by request, to protect their privacy.

Library of Congress Cataloging-in-Publication Data
McCutcheon, Paul, 1939–
  The new holistic way for dogs and cats : the stress-health connection/
Paul McCutcheon, and Susan Weinstein.
    p. cm.
  Includes bibliographical references and index.
  1. Pets—Diseases—Alternative treatment. 2. Pets—Effect of stress
on. 3. Holistic veterinary medicine. I. Weinstein, Susan, 1957– II.
Title.

  SF981.M285 2009
  636.089'55—dc22

2009012054

ISBN 978-1-58761-343-2

Printed in the USA

Cover and interior design by McGuire Barber Design
Photographs on title page and pages ix, 11, 39, 59, 61, 89, 119, 121,
155, 157, 181, and 211 © Michael Pettigrew

10 9 8 7 6 5 4 3 2 1

First Edition

This book is dedicated to you, the reader, who has taken the incentive to read this book. You are a special person who cares about your dog or cat's well-being. Your pet is lucky to have you.

Contents

PART ONE

Healing Concepts

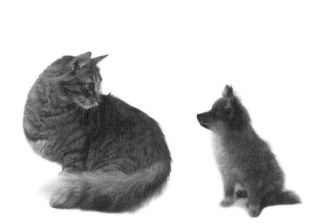

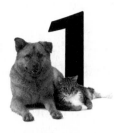

An Integrated Approach to Pet Care

When an aging Rottweiler called Liberty first walked into my clinic, her tragic past was years behind her. Surgery had helped repair her broken bones so she could live a normal life, and the people who adopted her after she was rescued made her life wonderful. But as she got on in years, arthritis set into her old injuries and she needed additional support that mainstream veterinary medicine could not provide. So her people, Maria and Catherine, brought the valiant old gal to me, hoping I might be able to offer her something more.

Years earlier, when she was three, Liberty had been thrown out of a moving van onto one of the busiest highways in North America. Although she broke a leg in the fall, the young Rottweiler managed to get off the road and run for hours before animal rescue workers finally tracked her down. When they found her, she was exhausted and confused.

According to the people who eventually adopted her, this extraordinarily gentle soul had been a junkyard dog who had been beaten, starved, and shot with a bullet in a futile attempt to make her vicious.

Her collar had torn her neck and she had cigarette burns in her mouth. This disturbing story made the front page of a major Toronto newspaper and was picked up by the media across both Canada and the United States. Liberty became a celebrity for Rottweiler rescue and other animal welfare organizations in North America and helped raise a lot of money for dogs in need. Donations also paid for the multiple surgeries she needed to wire together her fractured leg, remove the bullet still lodged in her body, and do emergency repair for the other physical damage she had suffered. When Maria Armstrong and Catherine Fogarty adopted her and took her home to join their other dogs and cats, they were committed to giving her the best life they could.

By the time she was nine, the dog's old knee injury had become arthritic, and her leg and back were also compromised. "It was something she developed over the years, and we had to take care of her," Maria says. Her people knew that steroids would ease her pain, but didn't want to risk that they might also make her need to urinate frequently. "She was a very proud dog. It really bothered her if she had an accident in the house, so we knew that steroids would be stressful for her in that way. Sometimes those things are necessary, but for Liberty we needed an alternative." That's when they brought her to me.

When she came in for her first appointment, Liberty held up her left hind leg and had difficulty walking. X-rays showed that she had broken a cruciate ligament in her knee. I had orthopedic surgeons discuss the options with Maria and Catherine, who decided against further surgery because the knee was already arthritic. Liberty was also severely obese, weighing in at 128 pounds, and had a thyroid condition. However, she was psychologically sound, according to Maria and Catherine, who said she was a sweetheart of a dog in spite of her background. My staff and I made it our goal to do everything within our capability to rehabilitate Liberty so that she could live out the rest of her days with the best possible quality of life.

To achieve this, we worked out a plan based on weight control, thyroid control, and joint therapy. We started her on glucosamine, chondroitin sulphate, and MSM (a natural anti-inflammatory) as well as antioxidants and a combination of herbal preparations. We also took over monitoring and fine-tuning her thyroid medications. Maria, Catherine, and I discussed how to improve Liberty's diet both for her overall wellness and to address her obesity. For the next three years, these measures enabled her to live reasonably well with her compromised knee.

After the old gal turned twelve, she started slowing down and was in obvious pain. Her arthritis was getting worse. So we added chiropractic treatments to the mix. Her mobility was sufficiently restored enough to carry her through comfortably until she passed on with dignity at age thirteen.

Liberty's story is a great example of how a deserving animal's life was given back to her by the reconstructive efforts of mainstream medicine, the supportive therapies of the holistic way, and the unfailing dedication of the people who loved her.

As your pet's human companion, you want to do the best you can for him or her, as do the clients who come to my clinic. This book will offer you better ways to do that. And whether or not you already use a holistic approach, it will give you new tools to ensure that your pet stays as happy and well as possible.

One of this book's most important tools involves learning a new perspective on health and healing—one that respects the best that natural health care and mainstream medicine have to offer, yet goes beyond the limitations of both. This new way of thinking will take you beyond fixing immediate problems and will give you a fresh and comprehensive take on prevention.

The holistic way of thinking also involves seeing your role and your veterinarian's role in a different way. Because you are the person closest to your dog or cat, you are in the best position to influence her well-being. You have the primary responsibility for making decisions that affect her quality of life. In my view, a veterinarian is a coach who provides expert opinions, perspectives, and advice about how to support your pet's wellness. At times, he may point you toward further resources and even toward other types of health care professionals to help you do that. Therefore, the information you find in these pages will also help you support your pet's wellness by updating your understanding of the relationship between you and your veterinarian in the holistic approach to pet care.

Finally, this book will endorse the value of various additional services that can help your dog or cat. In holistic veterinary care, paramedical services delivered by qualified professional acupuncturists, herbalists, chiropractors, homeopaths, and bioenergetic assessment technicians, to name a few, become a fundamental part of the total approach to maintaining wellness.

The holistic way of thinking that is so important to your pet's wellness begins with the way we look at health.

Holistic Health Care: More Than a Set of Treatments

Mainstream medicine has significantly influenced how people in the West think about health and healing. But since the 1970s, natural health care methods have steadily gained acceptance as effective, safe, and life-affirming ways to support the wellness of both humans and pets. These natural approaches are often referred to as holistic. In fact, the word *holistic* has picked up so much cultural momentum that it's used to sell products and services ranging from pet foods, shampoos, and beds to Sophie's weekly swim at the neighborhood dog spa. This encouraging sign shows that people want to do the best they can for their pets and the environment. But do all the claims that these products and services are holistic bear out?

For example, even the best foodstuffs can't be holistic (let alone natural) if most of the life has been cooked, dried, sanitized, and packaged out of them. Neither can a so-called herbal pet shampoo or grooming aid be completely wholesome and safe if it also contains industrial chemicals known to be harmful for a pet.

When it comes to health care, many people believe that a practice is holistic if it uses homeopathy, acupuncture, nutraceuticals, chiropractic, massage, or other natural therapies. But my clinical experience has taught me that no therapeutic remedy, supplement, or system is holistic in itself. **The holistic way cannot be defined by its remedies alone.** In fact, *any* therapy can serve either the goals of the holistic way or those of mainstream medicine. And those goals are very different.

WHAT IS THE *NEW* HOLISTIC WAY?

Based on more than four decades of veterinary practice, I want to take holistic health care into new territory. This is why I call my approach the *new* holistic way. I don't claim that all the ideas in this book are new. You will find many of them familiar if you already use modalities that are not part of mainstream medicine. Others have worked hard to promote these approaches, and I acknowledge that I am building on their excellent work. However, in my view many of these methods and concepts remain locked in and shaped by the historical contexts out of which they arose, as does mainstream medicine itself. Although they undoubtedly served well their original times, places, and cultures, today they are thrown together in a new context. As many different approaches to health care intermingle in this context, including traditional, indigenous, energy based, and recent developments in Western science, I see a synergy emerging.

To unleash this synergy, I offer a way of thinking that links the many different approaches to health care with our growing knowledge of how stress affects well-being. This is why I emphasized earlier that the new holistic way is not defined by its remedies alone. Instead, it guides us in choosing and applying whatever therapies or combination of therapies will work to address the health challenges that dogs and cats experience in contemporary life.

This new way of thinking is based on the premise that every expression of health—from wellness to unwellness to illness—emerges from the interaction of two factors. The first factor is the *living terrain*, which is the body itself, and the second is *stress*. I am convinced that better pet care will result when pet lovers and veterinarians understand that stress is the underlying cause of every form of health problem a dog or a cat can have.

In modern life, stress challenges the living terrain in infinite ways. Stress and the living terrain take part in a dynamic, never-ending dance from which all health outcomes flow. This book will help you choreograph this dance and lead your pet toward a more vibrant state of wellness.

By focusing on the relationship between stress and the living terrain, the new holistic way strives to achieve the following goals:

1. Support the health of the living terrain.
2. Free up blocked energy.
3. Consider the whole individual.
4. Look for the hidden stress factor that's causing the problem.
5. Adjust the environment to better meet the needs of the patient (the pet).
6. Use the solution that suits the individual best at the time.
7. Favor therapies that work *with* life's flow over those that work against it.

You will encounter these goals again and again throughout the pages of this book. In this chapter, we will focus on the first three goals.

The Living Terrain:
The Foundation of Wellness

Regardless of what may be the problem, when a client brings a pet into my clinic my aim is to help that animal thrive the way she is meant to. Nothing delights me more than seeing a dog or cat become radiant with enthusiasm for life, with shining eyes, glistening fur, a great appetite, and legs that move effortlessly with synchronicity and grace. My satisfaction as a veterinarian comes from helping my patients go from whatever condition they started with toward the highest degree of wellness they can attain.

The new holistic way begins and ends with supporting the condition of our pets' bodies—the living terrain.

In holistic thinking, wellness springs from the living terrain. Densely packed and highly complex, the living terrain consists of tissues that are made up of billions of living cells. The cells organize together to form organs, hormones, the nervous system—every part of the body—and from these, all the body's functions arise. Zooming in even closer for a moment, we can see that every cell is made up of molecules. Molecules are tiny bundles of energy—and energy is a superstar in the holistic view of life. We'll come back to the great importance of energy in a moment.

The living terrain is dynamic and *alive*. That's why I call it the *living* terrain. It has an integrity—an intelligence, we might say—of its own. It reaches for life just as a flower or tree reaches toward the sun. It constantly affects the environment of which it is a part, and the environment affects it in turn. All of us as individuals—whether canine, feline, or human—express ourselves through, and are one with, our own living terrain.

In a marvelously orchestrated and brilliant way, all aspects of a dog or cat's living terrain—its molecules, cells, tissues, organs, and systems—communicate and cooperate with each other to allow him to express himself according to his nature as a living being. We refer to this communication and cooperation between all aspects of the living terrain as synergy.

To support the health of the living terrain, the new holistic way focuses on all of these dimensions: the molecules, cells, tissues, organs, and systems; the synergistic communication among them; and the energy that manifests and powers them.

AN ANIMAL'S BODY IS HIS HOME

A helpful way of thinking about the body is to imagine that it's a little like a house. Of course, a living being can never be reduced to something that is not alive. But the comparison can help make some points.

If we think of a house as something that provides us with shelter and support for our daily lives, we think of more than the building. We also think of the systems and appliances that are included in the building, such as the furnace, oven, fridge, hot water tank, plumbing, washer and dryer, lighting, phones, computers, sound system, TV, and countless more. All of these things working properly and in harmony is what we think of as *home*—the life-supporting shelter that is much greater than the sum of its parts. This is an example of holistic thinking.

In the new holistic perspective, a truly healthy dog or cat will have all systems fully functioning in the home that is her body—her own living terrain. She will blossom with the fullness of life instead of experiencing pain, disability, or unhappiness. Her body will be in harmony with her surrounding environment, and that environment will be in agreement with what she needs. She will be in a state of homeostasis.

HOMEOSTASIS

Homeostasis means a state of balance or equilibrium. When harmony exists between the inner terrain and the outer environment, the body enjoys an ideal state of wellness. In other words, in holistic health care terms, homeostasis *is* wellness.

To once again liken the body to a house, a house is in balance when all systems run properly and work together to make everything happen as they're meant to happen. For example, the energy system powers the fridge, which keeps the food fresh, which nourishes the people who live in the house, who keep the energy system in good repair. This works like a continuous feedback loop. It's common in holistic thinking to envision a circle that replenishes itself—for better, when all is in harmony, or for worse, when something's amiss.

The new holistic way is based on the premise that all beings have the ability to heal themselves. This means that the body, or living terrain, of Fido, Fluffy, you, or me always wants to be in homeostasis. When invaders such as viruses, bacteria, or pollutants challenge homeostasis, the living terrain responds to protect itself. This self-protective aspect of the living terrain is what we call the immune system.

As the immune system tries to deal with a threat, it, along with the rest of the living terrain, will end up either stronger or weaker than it was before the threat came along. This outcome, in turn, will depend upon the degree of wellness it had available in the first place from which to respond to the stress. In other words, an immune system can only be as healthy as the body it protects and is a part of. (For more on how the immune system works, see page 52.)

This is why nourishing and supporting our pets' living terrains appropriately in everyday life is the single most important thing we can do for their wellness. (See Chapters 3 and 4 for general guidelines on how to do this.) Festus and Samson's health needs don't end the moment they leave my clinic. The new holistic way's number one priority is to keep the living terrain, including the immune system, as well as possible all the time. If Festus and Samson are bursting with wellness when they walk out the door to go home, they won't sustain that condition unless their people look after them in ways that allow their immune systems to remain strong. I consider it part of my job as a veterinarian to coach my clients about how to do that. You will find the kind of guidance I give in subsequent chapters of this book.

The Vital Importance of Free-Flowing Energy

The health of the immune system, like that of the rest of the living terrain, depends upon how well living energy flows through it. In the new holistic way, all paths lead back to the fundamental importance of energy.

THE WOUND THAT WOULDN'T HEAL

I first became aware of the role of energy flow to the living terrain's remarkable power to heal itself when I tried to help a German shepherd who had a bad leg wound that would not mend. Before I saw him, the dog had been taken to other clinics and been put through the gamut of mainstream therapies, including many different antibiotics. One dedicated vet even tried to surgically reestablish normal tissue in the area, after which the wound partially healed, but then it broke down and reopened again. When I saw it, it had formed a weeping, seeping, fistulous tract. There was no foreign object in it, no infection, no known reason why it wouldn't heal. But it would not.

Because I wanted to try stimulating the body's own ability to heal rather than using methods that acted directly upon the wound, I gave the shepherd an arbitrary dose of homeopathic Silicea tissue salts. Over a short period of time the wound healed up completely. I was thrilled to see a safe, subtle, natural substance such as this work so effectively.

I realized that the wound had not healed previously because the dog had an energy block that affected the area. Neither antibiotics nor surgery had done the trick; the fistula did not resolve until we used a therapy that removed the block on the subtle energy field. If we hadn't moved out the block, the healing would not have happened. Somehow, the homeopathic tissue salt enabled the healing process by releasing the block so that energy was able to flow freely again.

NOTHING HAPPENS WITHOUT ENERGY

Everything is made of energy, and energy powers everything. Nearly every ancient or traditional healing system has recognized this. Each tradition has its own understanding of where energy comes from and what it means. Whether they use the words chakras, chi, life force, spirit, or electrons, people are talking about energy. Whatever we may call it, free-flowing energy and the crucial role it plays are front and center in the new holistic approach to health care.

Looking through the lens of our Western mind-set, we have been slow to accept energy as a factor in health care. We think that if we can't see it, it isn't really there. Yet we accept other powerful forces that we can't see. For example, when was the last time you saw the wind? But we see and feel its tremendous effects as it bends trees, flaps the laundry on the line, pushes clouds around, or buffets the cars we ride in. It's the same with gravity. We don't *see* it, but we feel it and know it's really there. It's the reason we have to be careful climbing stairs and must hold pets or babies securely in our arms. As we age, we experience its effect on our bodies. Like the wind and gravity, the energy that moves us and forms our bodies really exists. We can't address our health needs if we ignore it or fail to acknowledge it.

Nothing happens without energy. The appliances that make a modern home comfortable depend upon its free and proper flow. When too little electricity flows, appliances slow down and grind to a halt. If too much electricity surges through them or flows in the wrong way, they short-circuit and malfunction or burn out altogether.

Like the electricity that flows through a house, the energy that flows through living beings keeps vital systems functioning at their best. An animal's health and well-being depend upon her life energy being able to flow as it's meant to. When her energy doesn't move well, physical problems begin to develop at the cellular level and interfere with the functions of tissues, organs, glands, and other crucial aspects of the body—as happened with the German shepherd whose wound would not heal. This is why holistic health care focuses on freeing up any blocked energy within a pet's living terrain.

In dogs, cats, and people, energy expresses itself not only physically but also emotionally and mentally. (The mental aspect is especially developed in humans.) Emotional and mental states affect the living terrain of our bodies, and the terrain, in turn, influences how we feel and think. Again, we see the wonderful synergy that manifests in each living being. When energy flows as it's meant to, our pets experience the balance of homeostasis. They feel the pleasure of life and the joy of good health. But when something blocks the physical or emotional energy that should flow through their living terrain, their wellness deteriorates. Then, signs and symptoms show up to tell us something is wrong.

But signs and symptoms manifest differently in every individual dog, cat, or human. This brings us to the next goal of the holistic way.

Taking Individuality into Account

Because signs and symptoms present themselves differently in everyone, the holistic way regards each patient as an individual who has a unique response to stressors that may challenge her living terrain.

TWO TERRIERS WITH IDENTICAL SYMPTOMS BUT DIFFERENT ILLNESSES

Sometimes two individuals will have the same illness and will display it in different ways. Other times, they will have different illnesses but show exactly the same symptoms. I had a chance to see this for myself when two dogs, both previously diagnosed with Cushing's disease, were brought to my clinic within a few weeks of each other.

The first case was that of a wire fox terrier called Casey who had typical signs of Cushing's and lab results that backed up the diagnosis. Cushing's disease involves overactivity of the adrenal gland and is often associated with a brain tumor affecting the pituitary gland. It typically reveals itself through excessive eating, drinking, fluid retention, and urination, and the patient becomes weak and lethargic. Because veterinarians don't yet know how to cure it, we try to control the condition and make the patient more comfortable for the time she has left. This is usually done using invasive pharmaceutical drugs that can have severe side effects.

Casey's people brought him to me because they'd been told that he had to be put on a drug that would have damaged his adrenal glands, and they didn't want to go that route. But there is another drug, used for treating Parkinson's disease in people, that will sometimes control Cushing's cases. I was hopeful it would work for Casey so we could avoid the other options. To the relief of my clients and me, it did work. With the help of the less risky pharmaceutical we were able to keep Casey going for a couple more years until he passed away.

The second case involved Rosie, an Airedale terrier who had the same symptoms as Casey. Even the lab reports of the two dogs matched. Rosie's people were aware of the standard Cushing's drugs and didn't want to risk her suffering their side effects, so before they agreed to use them they came to me, hoping for an alternative.

My first inclination was to approach Rosie's case the same way I had approached Casey's case. But as her people and I discussed her history, important information emerged. This dog was living under tremendous emotional stress. Josie and Rob were working out a marital separation, and they shared custody of Rosie by shifting her back and forth between them. As we talked, we realized that her symptoms became much worse when she stayed with Rob and eased off when she stayed with Josie. Something didn't add up—a dog would not have classic Cushing's disease in one environment but not in another. So, given Rosie's circumstances, I decided to try a different tack: we could experiment to see whether we could improve the dog's condition by reducing her environmental stress. At the same time, we would aid her living terrain with gentle, supportive remedies.

Josie and Rob agreed to try letting Rosie stay full time with Josie. I supplied them with raw adrenal supplements combined with appropriate herbs, as well as homeopathic and flower remedies. Once all these changes were in place, Rosie's symptoms completely disappeared.

I was delighted that we were able to solve such a challenging problem by modifying the environment instead of using powerful drugs. And it was evident that although Rosie's symptoms mimicked Casey's, she didn't have Cushing's at all. Instead, her adrenal glands were under stress induced by an emotional situation. If I'd looked solely at the similar signs and symptoms of the two cases, I would have treated them the same way and unnecessarily subjected Rosie to invasive drugs. The individual characteristics of these two dogs and their underlying circumstances made all the difference in the world.

When a pet's health deteriorates, the new holistic way guides us to focus on the aspects of her specific case. We consider her genetic background; her physical, environmental, social, and emotional history and present circumstances; and her particular signs or symptoms. Such information provides clues about the underlying cause of the patient's stress, as it did with Rosie. It also helps us gauge how her immune system has responded to the problem.

For example, *your* cat may display signs of an upper respiratory infection with a drippy nose and sneezing, in contrast to the cat next door, who responds to the same virus with a few minor sniffles. Your cat's individual signs reveal a lot, not only about which virus is attacking, but also about the kind of immune response she is able to mount against it. Taking note of each individual's distinct response also makes it possible to determine what kinds of support will be safe and appropriate for your particular pet at this moment in time.

The New Holistic Way and Mainstream Medicine

Supporting the living terrain, freeing up energy, and taking into account your dog or cat's individuality so we can see the distinct features of her response are goals of the new holistic way. These goals differ from those of mainstream medicine.

DIFFERENT WAYS TO THINK ABOUT HEALTH

Consider the way you think about health, be it your dog's, your cat's, or your own. When you think your pet isn't feeling well, what do you look for to help you decide what's wrong? How do you explain to yourself what you have found? How do you think these issues should be dealt with? Finally, what kind of outcome would convince you that you've solved your pet's problem? The way you answer these questions shows how you think about health and how this affects the health care choices you make. Likewise, the ways mainstream veterinarians and holistic veterinarians answer the same questions reveal how *they* think about health.

WHEN ABBOTT HAD EAR MITES

Before she became one of our clients, Jill had an unfortunate experience with Abbott, her mottled brown tabby cat. Abbott started having bouts where he would vomit, go off his food, and appear despondent. At first, Jill thought he might have developed a fur ball or eaten something that didn't agree with him, especially since he seemed to recover quickly on his own. Several months after these episodes began she noticed that he had ear mites. His fur became dull and greasy, and he began to lose weight. Jill took him to a nearby veterinary clinic.

Jill mentioned the cat's dull fur and occasional vomiting, but once the vet saw the ear mites he had no interest in these subtle symptoms. He identified the parasites as the problem and prescribed a pesticide-based drug for Abbott.

The ear mites did not go away, and Abbott's bouts of unwellness came more and more frequently. Jill took the cat to a second clinic, where she received a similar diagnosis and more pesticide-based drugs. This time the ear mites cleared up temporarily, but Abbott kept getting weaker and thinner and he vomited more often. His breath smelled offensive and he was clearly unhappy. He also began to urinate frequently.

Convinced there was something more than ear mites wrong with her cat, Jill sought a third opinion. The new vet noticed the ear mites but wanted to know about Abbott's history and was concerned to hear that he'd been vomiting, urinating frequently, and losing energy for months. She diagnosed him with chronic interstitial nephritis (chronic kidney inflammation), which she said he'd probably had for some time. Thinking more holistically than had her colleagues, she suggested that Abbott's long-term kidney problems may have led to the loss of condition that made him so vulnerable to ear mites. To her, persistent parasites were a sign of a more serious underlying problem, whereas Abbott's previous two vets had seen his stubborn infestation as the sole significant problem and had not considered them as a clue to a deeper illness.

Unfortunately, it was too late for Abbott. Repeated infection had destroyed most of his kidney tissue. Not only that, but pesticides and a questionable diet had handicapped his struggling organs even further. Had Abbott's subtle signs, symptoms, and history been considered sooner and in a broad and inclusive way, the stress on his kidneys may have been addressed before it led to permanent damage and he could have lived a happier, and probably longer, life.

Abbott's story illustrates important differences between the way mainstream medicine and the holistic way attempt to find out what's wrong when a pet is not well. In both approaches the veterinarian's first task is to look for signs and symptoms of the problem. Mainstream vets look at the pet's body for indications such as rashes, vomiting, diarrhea, or loss of appetite. They also look for physical changes that standard scientific tests can measure, such as temperature, white blood cell count, or the presence of antibodies. By contrast, holistic vets observe these same signs and physical changes but place them in a much larger framework. And because we consider the animal in the broadest possible context, we also look at physical, emotional, mental, and environmental factors that mainstream medicine has not traditionally taken into account. These include whatever is present for the pet in her current circumstances, including behavior, diet, activity level, mood, sleeping patterns, attitude, history of illnesses, surgeries, drugs or supplements, and recent life changes or tensions.

Once a veterinarian has identified the signs and symptoms of illness, he tries to find an explanation for them. Those guided by the mainstream perspective follow a reductionist way of thinking. That is, they see the part of the patient that shows symptoms as separate from the parts that don't. They pay attention to each organ, tissue, or cell in isolation, disconnected from the rest—just as Abbott's first two vets concerned themselves solely with his severely infected ears. Veterinarians who follow reductionist thinking see the patient's body as independent from his physical and emotional environment. The way all elements work together in synergy receives little, if any, attention. Although they may look for a cause such as a bacteria, gene, or parasite, their search often stops there because they regard the symptom itself— whether it be a rash, fever, tumor, or ear mites, as in Abbott's case—as the problem that must be solved. To solve these problems, they aim to match the symptoms to one of the disease categories that mainstream medicine has created for this purpose; this is what mainstream

Fighting Words or Healing Words?

The language that a health care approach uses gives us clues to the way of thinking that shapes it. For example, mainstream medicine uses competitive and military terms such as "fighting disease," "we'll beat this thing," "taking aggressive measures," "the battle against cancer," "curing" illness, or "succumbing" to it. It equates being healthy with being "not sick." In contrast, the holistic way uses terms that speak of harmony and realignment, such as "becoming whole again," "supporting the terrain," "freeing the energy," "restoring balance," and "encouraging healing." It equates being healthy with the presence of "wellness."

medicine means by diagnosis. Once the mainstream vet has matched the symptoms to a disease category, he develops a plan for fighting the disease, which he sees as the enemy.

In comparison, when searching for an explanation for signs and symptoms, veterinarians of the new holistic way are guided by holism as a way of thinking. Rather than narrowing the search, we widen it to the broadest context. We look for the connections between its many aspects and search through many levels for the underlying cause. For example, if a pet has symptoms of a virus, we consider not only the virus that challenged homeostasis but also the weakness in the living terrain that made her vulnerable to it. As well, we consider whether her environment might be undermining, rather than supporting, that terrain. We don't try to categorize symptoms into a disease we then have to fight. Instead, we let signs and symptoms point us to aspects of the pet's living terrain and her environment that might need to be strengthened or changed to support her return to wellness.

This leads us to the striking difference in the ways that mainstream medicine and the holistic approach use signs and symptoms to guide their respective plans of action. Because mainstream medicine sees signs and symptoms as manifestations of a disease that must be fought, the mainstream plan of action will focus on eliminating those signs and symptoms. This helps explain why in Abbott's case the first two vets focused on his ear mites as the primary problem, and then prescribed an insecticide to destroy them.

In the new holistic way, however, signs and symptoms play a powerful role as guideposts to other things. They draw our attention to a problem and give clues to its underlying cause. For instance, they may point to an energy blockage or a weakened immune system struggling to do its job, or they may tell us that the pet is facing an overwhelming health challenge—such as progressive kidney infection—that she can't meet without professional assistance. Additionally, signs and symptoms reveal how well the patient can handle the problem and is responding to the support we're trying to give. Therefore, they guide us in helping her to return to homeostasis—to wellness.

Mainstream medicine and the holistic way also differ in how they relate to natural processes. The mainstream approach to treating health problems tends to interfere with natural processes instead of working with them. Because its plan of action is to attack symptoms, it often shuts down the immune system or damages vital organs as a collateral result. For instance, veterinarians see a lot of animals who are bothered by seasonal allergies. These pets typically present with inflamed and itchy skin. To relieve the animal's discomfort, mainstream medicine would typically prescribe prednisone, a steroid, to suppress the symptoms. But unfortunately, steroids also weaken the immune system, and a weak immune system can lead to problems far more serious than allergies. For example, a strong immune system controls cancerous and other abnormal cells. When suppressed, it is less able to perform its functions. So while a suppressed immune system doesn't *cause* cancer, its compromised ability to deal with abnormal cells allows them to develop more freely.[1]

Veterinarians also commonly see pets who are diagnosed with cancer. A vet who follows a mainstream approach may administer chemotherapy to kill the malignant cells. But these drugs can also brutally damage the pet's immune system, which may have already been compromised before her cell growth went out of control. In my experience, chemotherapy is most effective when it is most invasive. Its side effects may cause an animal great suffering, sometimes worse than the cancer itself might cause, and may even kill her. Mainstream medicine's goals are to save or prolong life whenever possible—sometimes without taking into account whether this is best for the patient. It will find and destroy the culprits that cause disease, but it will also suppress functions that enhance the patient's enjoyment of life, while hoping that the body will somehow return to normal.

In the holistic way, we approach a health problem by focusing on the patient's individual combination of symptoms, whether or not they fit into a recognized profile. We pay careful attention to the condition of her living terrain and her environment, and we read her symptoms as clues about the bigger picture to which her living terrain is responding. When we devise a plan to support her healing, or, if she cannot fully recover, a plan of palliative care to ease her suffering, we take into account as many factors as possible. With each new case, the holistic veterinarian investigates what is going on in *this* individual's body, environment, and lifestyle. We recognize that the living terrain always seeks homeostasis, and that, given the right assistance, the body will attempt to heal itself not only from cuts and broken bones but also from harder-to-solve conditions such as cancer or arthritis. In the holistic way, we work *with* the body and its natural processes to solve a problem. And although we try to relieve uncomfortable symptoms, we do not suppress them, because we see signs and symptoms as guideposts: they tell us what's wrong, whether we're on the right track, and how well the patient is recovering.

Finally, mainstream medicine and the new holistic way also differ in how they determine that a health problem has been solved. Mainstream medicine considers its job done once signs and symptoms disappear.

The new holistic way, on the other hand, believes a pet has achieved optimal wellness not when signs and symptoms have disappeared but when she radiates good health. It also recognizes that in the early stages of recovery, a pet may have a healing crisis in which her symptoms get *worse* before they get better. In fact, a temporary worsening of symptoms may mean that the immune system has strengthened its response to a challenge. Even after a crisis has passed and symptoms have disappeared, a holistic veterinarian may not consider the problem solved. Instead, he may provide long-term support if the crisis revealed that the condition of the pet's living terrain or the environment in which she lives are unhealthy and may not improve.

WORSENING SYMPTOMS MAY BE A STAGE IN RECOVERY

Sometimes an animal who has been given a homeopathic remedy or other therapy that supports the living terrain goes into a healing crisis before she improves. I witnessed a thrilling example of this with a cat who, like Abbott, was also in the late stages of kidney failure, but whose outcome was markedly different.

As cats get older their kidneys often start to degenerate, and Littlebit was a typical case. By the time I saw the black domestic short-haired cat, he was dehydrated and had major weight loss, weakness, and anemia. He had improved temporarily after receiving therapy at another clinic, but when he took a turn for the worse his people had been advised that he should be euthanized. It's often appropriate to think about euthanasia at a time like this, but his people weren't ready for it. They also didn't want to have him hospitalized again because it was very stressful for him. Hoping there might be another answer that would keep him going at least for a while, they brought him to me.

When I first laid eyes on Littlebit, I could see he was in really bad shape. I concurred with his original diagnosis of kidney failure, and I made sure the clients understood that although we could try a few things, they should be prepared not to see any improvement. I gave Littlebit high-potency homeopathic Carbo Vegetalis, Arsenicum Album, and Nat Mur to generate some metabolic response within his system and detoxify his kidneys, and I sent him and his people home with a needle and bag of subcutaneous fluids so they could administer it to him themselves.

That evening at home, Littlebit appeared to go sharply downhill. He looked so ill that his people thought he was going to die overnight, and I wouldn't have been surprised if he had. But the next morning they were amazed to find him up and eating. When they phoned to tell me this they were very excited. I was especially pleased, because I had not expected him to respond so well.

I always love to get a phone call like this. This cat was either going to die or rejuvenate, and something stimulated him to come back to life. I'm not too concerned to figure out which remedy did what; most important to me is that somehow homeopathy helped him heal himself. For many months after this Littlebit maintained a reasonable quality of life before he finally passed away.

To me, this is what veterinary medicine is all about. It's very gratifying to be able to give support and get a response in a very touch-and-go case such as Littlebit's.

The Gifts of Mainstream Medicine

Although mainstream medicine's overall approach does not meet all our pets' health needs, I believe that careful use of mainstream methods may, in certain circumstances, be the most holistic choice to help a particular pet. They are sometimes just what we need. Mainstream diagnostic tools such as blood tests, tissue biopsies, or X-rays, and its treatment modalities such as surgery, pharmaceutical drugs, and radiation tend to be dramatic and invasive, and while this is their weakness,

Izzie and Ozzie

Let's say that Izzie has a rapidly growing skin cancer, and Ozzie is rushed into the clinic with internal injuries due to an accident. Neither of these pets may have enough time to regain homeostasis before these overwhelming health threats take them down. In cases like these, aggressive modalities, skilfully applied, may buy them enough time to heal themselves after all. For example, surgery can remove Izzie's cancer before it gets any worse, and it can reconstruct Ozzie's damaged tissues enough to help him hold his own until his body begins to recover.

Anesthetics will spare them the pain of the surgery, and other drugs, given intravenously, will help stabilize them immediately afterward. Surgery and drugs are designed to save lives in exactly these situations.

But invasive modalities should only be used when they serve holistic goals. After we've dealt with an immediate danger, we must tailor an individual plan to nourish each pet's living terrain and enhance his return to the highest possible level of wellness. This will likely include short- or long-term dietary changes, plus the use of subtler modalities such as homeopathy, Reiki, or acupuncture. For Izzie, we'd look at which stressful factors may have preceded his cancer to see whether we can improve his environment. For Ozzie, we'd want to find out what circumstances led to his accident to try to prevent a similar event in the future.

in the right situations it is also their strength. Mainstream medicine shines in the following areas.

EMERGENCY INTERVENTIONS

Emergency interventions may involve anything from first aid in the case of life-threatening injuries to the speedy removal of aggressive cancerous growths. They can save a life in crisis and can allow more time for modalities that work *with* the living terrain to support the body

Two Different Kinds of Specialists

The different frameworks of mainstream medicine and the new holistic way create different kinds of experts. The holistic veterinarian often becomes qualified in many therapeutic methods. For example, a holistic vet who is trained to perform surgery and prescribe pharmaceutical drugs may also become a homeopath, an acupuncturist, and a nutritionist, or qualify in other therapies. On the other hand, mainstream medicine's tendency to study elements in isolation has led it to create specialists who concentrate on one narrowly defined field of health and rarely look for connections to other realms—often, not even to the realms of other mainstream specialists. The refined, exclusive focus of the medical specialist is exactly the opposite from the all-inclusive viewpoint of the holistic veterinarian.

to return to homeostasis and the best possible wellness. For example, if a pet has an aggressive cancer, without surgery she may not have enough time for a radical change in diet and supportive modalities to help her shift toward homeostasis. In such a case, immediate surgical removal of the growth may stop the cancer's progress long enough to allow other holistic measures to take effect.

PAIN RELIEF AND PALLIATIVE CARE

Pain relief can be a great compassion. For example, a dog with arthritis who no longer responds to measures that support the living terrain, such as glucosamine or traditional Chinese herbs, will live with chronic pain that will only get worse over time. For such a dog, carefully chosen pain relief can provide a better quality of life. Still, it's not always best to suppress pain. For example, a dog will favor a sore, sprained leg and give it a chance to recover, whereas if the pain has been dulled the dog may use the leg as though there's nothing wrong and cause permanent damage. But when suffering is chronic or severe, as is the case immediately after surgery or an accidental injury, the kindness of pain relief is one of the great gifts of mainstream medicine.

Once again, a health care approach cannot be defined by its treatments alone. Almost any healing modality can be used in accordance with either the holistic or the medical approach. For example, if we clear up symptoms with homeopathy (a modality usually associated with holistic practice) but we don't look for the conditions that prompted those symptoms in the first place, we are practising in accordance with mainstream medicine's goals. To approach the problem holistically, we need to address the deeper issue with a change in diet or lifestyle or other ways of supporting the living terrain and correcting the environment to better suit the pet's needs. In the same way, although it's not holistic to treat back pain by doing no more than supplying drugs for pain relief, in my view it *is* holistic to give pain-relieving drugs when measures such as chiropractic care and glucosamine supplements can no longer sufficiently support an individual's quality of life.

VETERINARIANS ARE INDIVIDUALS, TOO

Before we move on, I want to make a final point about mainstream medicine and the new holistic way. Although veterinarians tend to subscribe to the ways of thinking in which they trained, we are still individuals and shouldn't be categorized solely by the modalities we use. For example, some vets who employ modalities such as homeopathy and acupuncture may use them to achieve mainstream medicine's more short-term goals of ending the body's uncomfortable symptoms instead of dealing with the symptoms' underlying cause.

Likewise, some vets who use drugs and surgery as their primary modalities may take into account a broader range of factors such as environment and emotional state when trying to find the cause of a pet's problem. They may also, at least as a first step, recommend measures that support the living terrain, such as dietary changes or nutritional supplements, in hope of avoiding drugs or surgery. But these vets will typically rely upon drugs, surgery, and radiation, rather than a wider holistic repertoire, for two reasons.

First, they've been trained to use them and probably feel most secure with them. Second, in many jurisdictions, especially in the United States and Canada (it's different in Europe and many other places), mainstream doctors are not allowed to use tools that have not emerged from the mainstream medical tradition. Fortunately for our pets, veterinarians are often allowed more scope than medical doctors who deal with human patients, and may use both mainstream and living terrain-supporting modalities in their practices.

The Health Care of the Future

Clearly, whether we support our pets' health care holistically depends not so much on which modalities we choose—or whether we buy natural products, for that matter—but on why and how we use them and what we hope to achieve with them. And while both natural and mainstream medical tools have a place in holistic practice, the mainstream way of thinking about health leads to a very limited approach to health care. By thinking holistically, we can assess situations more broadly, choose tools more wisely, and have greater success in restoring homeostasis. In my experience, only the holistic way can fully support an animal's optimal wellness.

Knowing the difference between the mainstream approach and the new holistic way provides you with a valuable tool for making crucial decisions about the care of your dog or cat. The next chapter will provide you with a second valuable tool: the understanding that stress is the underlying cause of every health problem a dog or cat can have.

ENDNOTES

1. Donna F. Kusewitt and Laura J. Rush, "Neoplasia and Tumor Biology," in *Pathological Basis of Veterinary Disease, 4th edition,* eds. M. Donald McGavin and James F. Zachary, 253–298 (St Louis: Mosby Elsevier 2007); Theresa L. Whiteside, "Immune Suppression in Cancer: Effects on Immune Cells, Mechanisms and Future Therapeutic Intervention," *Seminars in Cancer Biology* 16, no. 1 (2006): 3–15.

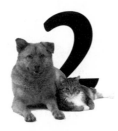

Stress: The Key to Animal Wellness

Cory, an intense little terrier, came into my office with a pink rash on his flank. Karina, his person, had given the rash a little time but it didn't clear up by itself, so she brought Cory in to see me. The little guy chewed and licked at his skin, making the rash worse.

Karina said she had no idea what might be causing the problem. For example, Cory had no contact with caustic chemical cleaners or pesticides. And he'd never before shown signs of allergies, which dogs tend to express through their skin. This was Cory's first rash.

When I asked Karina whether there had been any recent changes in Cory's living situation that might cause him emotional stress, she mentioned that she and her husband had just had their first baby. I said this may be the clue we were looking for. First, under even the best conditions, pregnancy can be stressful for a woman, and her dog would pick up on that. So Cory's stress may have begun before the child was born. And once the baby came, from Cory's point of view it was a new member born into the pack. In other words, he had become insecure about his place in his world. Insecurity about place in the pack is a primal source of anxiety for a dog. Karina said this made sense because Cory had been with her since before she met her husband, so he may have felt progressively displaced as her husband and then the baby joined the scene.

Emotional stress can express itself in both behavioral and physical changes, depending on the weaknesses a dog may have in his system. Cory was probably predisposed toward developing allergies, and the stress of the baby's arrival caused him to manifest this in a rash. To help him adapt to his expanding family, Cory needed the bond with his people to be strengthened, to be reassured that his place among them was secure. So I recommended that Karina make sure he got a share of her time every day. Her husband, too, should take a bigger role with the dog, involving him in activities such as extra walks to keep him occupied. We could offer Cory additional support such as flower remedies customized to his individual requirements, but for his condition to resolve his underlying stress had to be reduced.

It worked. Karina and her husband made sure Cory got more focused, positive attention every day, and eventually his rash cleared up.

Because both holistic and mainstream practice have become more accepting of emotional stress as a health factor, a veterinarian of either persuasion might deduce that stress had led to Cory's rash. A mainstream thinker would still see the rash itself as the problem and would probably provide steroids and maybe antibiotics to suppress it. But a holistic thinker would look for the problem's deeper underlying cause, and then would approach the problem from more than one angle. Working from the belief that the body wants to return to homeostasis, she might suggest supportive therapies to strengthen the pet's living terrain and flower remedies to soothe his anxiety while also thinking of ways that his stress could be relieved.

Cory's case shows how emotional stress can relate to a physical ailment. But stress plays a greater role than many people think in the well-being of cats and dogs. This chapter will show you why I'm convinced that stress is the sole cause of *everything* that happens to our pets' health.

In the dynamic dance of wellness, stress is the eternal challenger to the living terrain, which must constantly respond to it. It's the universal factor that lies behind not only illness but also its opposite pole, wellness, and the whole spectrum of *un*wellness that stretches between the two. (See Chapter 5 for more about assessing unwellness.) The more we understand about stress in a dog or cat's life, the better we can manage it so that he can thrive in the way he's meant to.

To manage a pet's stress well, we need to get past some common misconceptions. Mass media and advertising often represent stress as though it is solely a negative emotional or psychological response to the pressures of life. Although this is part of the truth, it makes up only a small aspect of what stress means to wellness.

What Is Stress?

In my veterinary practice, I use the concept of stress that scientist and medical doctor Hans Selye originally developed for humans in the 1970s. Selye defined stress as *the body's nonspecific response to demands from the environment around it.* Today, we understand that stress comes from causes both inside and outside ourselves, because our bodies are also part of the environment in which we live—an environment that's not only physical but also emotional, energetic, and mental. By expanding Selye's concept of stress and applying it to pet care, we open up new possibilities for supporting our pets' natural impulses toward wellness.

These new possibilities include therapies from both physically based and energy-based approaches to health care. (See Chapter 7 on the different approaches, beginning on page 161.) That's because the concept of stress grounds our understanding of energy in physical science. We might say that an animal's response to stress happens at the point where his energy—or life-force—expresses itself physically

41

Normal Stress Is a Part of Life

In the dog park, all kinds of interactions take place. For instance, Mollie and Saba are good friends who play hard together until they are tired. While they are romping one day, Bruiser enters the scene. A territorial fellow, Bruiser likes to strut about for a while before he lets his hair down with the other dogs. Saba, more highly strung than Mollie, stops playing and keeps an eye on Bruiser until he settles down while Mollie remains more relaxed and tries to prompt Saba to play again. Nearby, Dingo the retriever loves nothing more than to chase a ball or stick, but Jellybaby, a competitive large brown mix, growls threateningly at Dingo because he wants to claim the stick. Snowflake and Glacier, two Huskies, love to run far away from their person, who shouts after them to come back. This concerns Baron, who hails from a herding breed, so he rounds up the wayward Huskies and brings them back time and again. As long as the stress in the park doesn't become overwhelming, most of the dogs enjoy and benefit from the socializing and exercise they get there. Reasonable stress is part of life.

through the animal's quality of health. By taking stress as our starting point for looking at wellness, we can embrace both body-based and energy-based approaches to health care. In other words, the stress perspective does not force us to choose between physical versus energy-based theories about health. Rather, it has room for both.

In spite of its reputation for being negative, stress in itself is neither bad nor good. In one form or another, people and animals deal with it all the time. Part of being alive means encountering a never-ending parade of factors that create stress. Hans Selye called these *stressors*, and they involve every kind of life-need a dog or cat can have, from clean, fresh air, to correct climate, to appropriate diet, to emotional security, to mental stimulation—you name it. An animal's potential for wellness depends upon how well he can respond to stress at any given moment.

HOW STRESS CONTRIBUTES TO WELLNESS

As a dog or cat moves through life, stress constantly challenges him. The pet responds by trying to maintain, or regain, homeostasis in whichever ways he can. His wellness will *increase* if he can draw from his own living terrain enough energy to respond strongly, and if the stressor he faces is appropriate for him as a species and as an individual. This is the role stress plays in creating wellness.

For example, let's see how Angus and Mindy, a healthy dog and cat, respond to stress by becoming more well. One pleasant afternoon, Angus enjoys a game of fetch with Dave, his human companion. Eventually, the stress of all the running and chasing tires him out. To restore homeostasis, which in Angus's case means to calm his heart rate, cool down, and give his muscles a chance to recover, he lies down to rest and pant. Or take Mindy, a short-haired cat who finds herself prowling outside on a bitterly cold winter night. Soon, the stress of the cold threatens to dangerously lower her body temperature. To maintain homeostasis—which in this case means to keep from freezing—Mindy gives up the hunt and joins her people in the house where it's warm.

After Angus has taken a break and Mindy has spent some time snuggled next to the radiator, they both recover their balance. Fresh energy has renewed their bodies and spirits. Angus wants to get up to play again, and Mindy wants to resume hunting. Both are interested in life, and want to return to activities that fulfill their needs.

Angus and Mindy show what it looks like when stress recharges a pet's energy and increases his or her wellness. When stress leads to a happy and healthy outcome, we call it *positive* stress.

DISTRESS: WHEN STRESS BECOMES A PROBLEM

However, a cat or dog who isn't able to respond well to a stressor loses homeostasis and, therefore, his wellness. For example, Cyrus, a white domestic long-haired cat, and his buddy, a gray tabby named Marble, moved with Joey, their person, into a basement apartment. The new place was small and afforded the cats no opportunity to exercise. Soon, Cyrus started to develop urinary infections, but Marble, the tabby, was fine. We put Cyrus on herbal urinary tract cleansers and homeopathics, which seemed to clear up the infections temporarily but never resolved them completely. Then we tried antibiotics, but had the same results. Joey and I agreed that Cyrus's trouble must be related to the move and would correct itself once he adjusted. But when it kept coming back, we looked at specific environmental factors that could be the underlying cause.

Cats are vulnerable to a change of environment, although individuals vary in their ability to handle it. In this case, it appeared that Cyrus couldn't cope with this type of stress as well as Marble could. He showed his distress in a common feline weak spot—the urinary tract. Cyrus needed extra support to adapt to his new environment.

As Joey and I discussed the possibilities, I suggested he try exercising the cats out in the hall, because the apartment didn't provide enough room. They should be given fun things to do out there, such as balls to bat around and catnip toys or laser beams to chase. Most important, Joey himself should be out there playing with them.

Joey set aside time to play with the cats in the hall every day, and the plan worked. With the extra attention and tender loving care they received, along with the physical exercise, Cyrus's infections stopped.

Loss of homeostasis tends to show up first as the subtle malaise of *unwellness*. (See Chapter 5.) Unwellness usually manifests in signs that don't register in mainstream medicine's diagnostic tests, although if we're well attuned to our pets we may sense it anyway. If a pet can't resolve his unwellness on his own—in other words, if the stressor gets the upper hand over his living terrain—he will become *ill*. Unlike unwellness, illness produces physical changes that standard medical tests can measure. These may include a spike in temperature, an increase in white blood cells, and so on, and it's upon this kind of

Speaking of Stress . . .

Although stress can have positive and negative effects, this book emphasizes the need to reduce as much negative stress as we possibly can for our pets' optimal wellness. To make communication easier, whenever I talk about getting rid of stress and don't specify which type, I'm talking about negative stress.

evidence of illness that mainstream medicine bases its diagnoses and treatments. (See Chapter 1.) In stress language, when a pet becomes significantly physically ill we say he is in *distress*. This differs in human terms, when saying that someone is distressed usually means that she's worried or anxious.

Stress that leads to greater wellness is positive. Stress that depletes energy and leads to unwellness or illness is negative. Negative stress causes every problem our pets may have in life, whether physical, emotional, or mental. As we learn how to manage our pets' stress, their physical, emotional, and mental states of being will become much more positive overall.

Every creature is born with a different capacity to respond to stress. A pet with a stronger stress response mode will recover more quickly and completely than one with a weaker stress response mode, even if they both have the best health care and environmental support. As I explained in Chapter 1, the energy our pets draw from their living terrain determines the strength of their ability to respond. Understanding an animal's stress response mode helps us understand when he really needs help and which types of supportive measures he should have. (See pages 171–179.) But no matter what kind of constitution he is born with, every pet can be helped to respond better than he did.

How stress affects the health of our pets is complicated, and it involves some awesome physical processes. Knowing the gist of these processes—and their all-important relationship to the energy flow that keeps our four-legged friends alive—gives us the scientific basis for understanding how stress affects a dog or cat's well-being.

The Physical Facts of Stress

Dogs, cats, and humans share many physiological systems that serve to keep us alive. Two major systems are the stress response system[1] and the immune system.[2] Let's take a quick look at them.

THE STRESS RESPONSE SYSTEM

When Jake, a German shepherd-husky cross, encounters stress, here in a general sense is what happens. Jake's stressor could be an emotional challenge relating to his circumstances such as another animal entering his territory, a physical challenge such as being pursued by a swarm of deer flies, or a cellular challenge such as unfriendly bacteria. Depending on the nature of the stressor, Jake will either:

- Avoid it. For example, picture Jake pounding at the door, asking to be let in where the deer flies can't torment him.
- Compete with it. For example, Jake's body raises its own temperature to drive out unfriendly viruses.
- Cooperate with it. For example, Jake senses that the new dog next door is more of a friend than an enemy.[3]

Whatever his reaction, Jake's nervous system, hormone-producing glands, and organs all get in on the act. First, he becomes aware of the challenge. If it confronts him in the outer world, he becomes aware of it consciously. If it confronts him within his body at the cellular level, special chemical substances such as cytokines communicate the threat to his stress response system.

Next, his nervous system produces special hormones such as adrenaline and the steroid cortisol. His immune system's cells have built-in receptors for these stress hormones. In turn, they speed up

Energy and Stress

Every aspect of wellness and illness flows back to the relationship between energy and stress. Ancient approaches to health care, plus some of the newer ones, are based in various ways upon this awareness. That's why they work.

Jake's heart rate and respiratory function, make him more mentally alert, and prepare his muscles to exert themselves as required. From the moment he first perceives a stressor, his entire being quickens. It's as though he has physiologically put his foot on the accelerator pedal.

As Jake responds to the stressor, he draws upon the energy that his cells provide. During this heightened activity, his cells also create potentially destructive by-products that his body will deal with after the emergency has passed. But first, he has to deal with the stressor itself.

As long as he has to deal with the stressor, his nervous system and his stress hormones give each other signals about when and how much to increase his response to it. If he has enough energy and his living terrain is strong, and provided the stressor is one that his species has evolved to deal with, he'll be able to resolve his stress by removing himself from it, vanquishing it, or accepting and coexisting with it.

THE NEED FOR REST AND RECOVERY

Once Jake has dealt with the stressor, his body puts on the brakes. His nervous system sends out other hormones to counteract the response that it had earlier fired up. As a result, Jake stops producing stress hormones, and his heart rate, respiration, muscle tension, and brain activity calm down.

Once he has come out of his stress response state, Jake needs time to rest. While he does so, his cells will repair themselves and replenish

How Dogs Respond to New Situations

According to highly respected Canadian dog behavior expert Silvia Jay, most dogs are not born confident, so they approach each new situation with caution. When confronted with a social or an emotional stressor, such as a new dog next door, a dog's pupils will dilate and he will briefly hesitate before he responds. This momentary withdrawal enables him to increase his social distance from the stressor until it becomes more predictable in his mind. If he is not permitted to withdraw or else continues to perceive the stressor as unpredictable, he will then likely try to compete with it. Competing may also be learned behavior; dogs who have learned to compete before sizing up a situation will respond this way first instead of withdrawing. Finally, once a dog is confident that a stressor is not a threat, he will cooperate with it. For example, he may befriend the dog next door or agree to peacefully coexist in close proximity with him. (See the Selected Bibliography in the Appendix.)

their energy supply for next time. His body now deals with any harmful by-products, such as lactic acid and free radicals, that his cells may have created while he was under stress.[4]

A pet must always have ample time to recover after responding to a stressful challenge. If Jake doesn't get the relief that he needs—in other words, if the stress is too intense or prolonged and he loses more energy than he can recoup—he'll end up with cell or tissue damage that will be harder to repair. He'll build up more destructive by-products, such as free radicals, than he can cope with, and he will become vulnerable to the negative health effects these may cause. And if his energy continues to drain, he'll be weaker when he has to cope with stress in the future. In other words, he'll lose homeostasis and head down the road toward unwellness and illness. The downward spiral can be initiated either by acute stress that's too severe or by chronic, long-term stress.

THE DIFFERENCE BETWEEN ACUTE STRESS AND CHRONIC STRESS

A six-year-old yellow Lab named Billy ate a cup of raisins one day and began vomiting shortly thereafter. He lost his appetite and appeared to be depressed and in pain. His people rushed him to a veterinary emergency clinic, where laboratory work revealed that he had suffered acute renal failure. Raisins are an environmental toxin for some dogs, and they were the likely cause of Billy's crisis. He was in acute distress and it wasn't clear whether he would survive.

Billy remained in intensive care for two weeks and a specialist took over his case. He was put on intravenous therapy during which he began to urinate more often and his appetite returned. Finally, he was taken off the IV and sent home, but then his improvement stalled and he went downhill again. His people brought him to my clinic a few days later. Three weeks had passed since he'd eaten the raisins.

We switched Billy to a homemade, sardine-based diet. We added lots of omega-3 oils, plus other supportive therapies such as probiotics, organotherapy supplements, and chlorophyll to detoxify and improve his pH level. Then we added homeopathic drainage remedies for his kidneys. Billy gradually improved.

A month later, we modified the homeopathics and adjusted his diet. The anemia resolved and he seemed to be doing well, but tests showed that his kidney levels were still problematic. Although his test results were discouraging, experience has taught me not to make a judgment call about an animal's condition based strictly on laboratory results, but to take into account how he appears to be feeling. Billy appeared to be feeling significantly better than his kidney levels would suggest. So we kept on with the diet and the drainage remedies.

It was a long haul, but Billy's kidney levels slowly improved and after seven more months of supportive therapy they stabilized at last. I was very relieved. We had finally achieved what we had set out to do and brought this dog back from acute distress to satisfactory physiological function.

As it was with Billy, acute stress is immediate and intense. It can be caused by an accident, a sudden infection, or a powerful toxin. Although it's usually short-lived, if it's too much for our pets to handle, it can have very serious consequences. But if a pet is healthy, she will overcome most acute stressors. You can help your pet by preventing acute stress in whatever ways you are able and by supporting her living terrain so that if a challenge confronts her, she can successfully hold her own.

Chronic stress, on the other hand, can be a real drag on wellness. Often, when a dog or cat with a serious illness such as cancer is brought to my clinic, I will discover that she has been suffering from chronic stress due to a long-standing cause that had been neither identified nor addressed.

For example, a client once told me about a German shepherd named Sojourner who belonged to a friend of hers. The friend was rarely satisfied with others' behavior, including her dog's. German shepherds are highly responsive and live to please their people, but Sojourner could never please her person. Instead, every nuance of her behavior was subject to her human companion's attempts to change it in some way. Sojourner became increasingly nervous, barking at the slightest provocation, and eventually her person purchased an electric collar that would shock her whenever she barked, a solution I would never advocate.

The collar had little effect on the barking, but it confused Sojourner, who became even more anxious, thus intensifying her chronic stress. In the prime of her life, Sojourner developed cancer and died. Interestingly, her person also died of cancer not long afterward. I am not implying that the electric collar caused the dog's cancer, but I am saying that I have seen a lot of cases where a seriously ill pet endured chronic emotional stress for a long time before the illness developed. I am convinced there is a connection between long-term emotional stress and cancer.

Raisins Can Be Dangerous to Dogs

Raisins and grapes are an environmental toxin to some dogs, in whom they cause kidney failure. Lots of dogs eat raisins and don't respond badly; it depends on the individual. But the possibility exists that a dog may react in this way. Raisins are but one food that dogs and cats should not eat. See The Stress-Busters Diet for Dogs and Cats in the Appendix for a list of others.

Fortunately, not all cases of chronic stress have such a tragic outcome, and I certainly don't mean to suggest that if your dog or cat has endured chronic stress he will end up with cancer. Once a stressor is recognized and modified and the living terrain given support, a pet will improve either emotionally or physically or both, and at least some future problems will be prevented. But because of the toll chronic stress takes on the living terrain, many of these pets will need ongoing support to maintain their best level of wellness. It's worth the effort—it's wonderful to see a pet who has suffered from chronic stress become both happier and healthier.

Because it is prolonged and persistent, chronic stress can wear down a pet over time. Its effects manifest differently in each individual. One animal may show it through a behavioral issue; another, through a gastrointestinal disturbance; and a third, through unexplained weight loss. It may also produce problems with organs or glands, such as heart disease or diabetes. Chronic stress tends to need ongoing support, but the right approach will ease, and sometimes even resolve, the health care issues it may cause.

Chronic stress can also compromise a pet's health indirectly. For example, she may become more susceptible to infections, and eventually to degenerative conditions such as cancer or allergies. These conditions often vary in intensity. For instance, allergies tend to come and go depending on the season or the availability of irritants; arthritis is affected by damp weather or too much or too little exercise, and cancerous growths don't always grow at a steady rate and sometimes actually get smaller. Although appropriate health care will improve most of these problems, they can be very challenging to address. All of them depend on the strength of the other major factor that plays a starring role in maintaining our pets' health: the immune system.

THE IMMUNE SYSTEM

The first time an opportunistic stressor such as a virus, unfriendly bacteria, parasite, or toxin tries to enter your dog or cat's living terrain, a sequence of chemical communications tells the immune system about the problem. The immune system responds with helpers such as white blood cells (leukocytes) that attack the invader and drive it back. Once the immune system has successfully rid the living terrain of a stressor, it also creates a tag for that particular stressor so that it can mark and recognize it in the future and react more quickly. Tags also help it tell the difference between invaders (not self) and the living terrain (self). Once the immune system tags an invader, we call it an *antigen*. If the same stressor dares to show up again, the immune system recognizes it and deals with it as quickly and effectively as possible. We call this *immunity*.

If the invaders are resistant, the immune system turns up the heat—sometimes literally—to drive them out. When a client rushes into my clinic because her cat has a high fever, I reassure her that this is a good sign—the immune system is working and it's doing what it's supposed to do. Fever is only one example of the immune system protecting the terrain. There are many others, including inflammation, mucus discharge, vomiting, diarrhea, and so on. Pus, made of dead white blood cells that have spent themselves trying to kill bacteria that got into a wound, is a great illustration of the immune system at work. Signs from the immune system also serve as a burglar alarm, announcing that

The Importance of Joy

As animal lovers, we know that dogs and cats are both physical and emotional beings. They delight in the loving, focused attention we give them; in exercise that makes them feel wonderfully alive; in having time every day for fun and play with you or others of their own kind. Dogs in particular must have a sense of a responsibility or role to play to help look after the household pack. There's no such thing as having too much joy.

something has invaded the pet's living terrain. Mainstream medicine sees these symptoms as the problems to be solved, whereas a holistic vet would read them as signals that a pet's immune system *is* responding to a threat and *how* it is responding to the threat.

When the immune system is healthy, its chemical messengers warn it about threats, and it creates inflammations and discharges and produces enough white blood cells to drive out invaders. It makes sure that normal, everyday cell divisions stay within balanced and acceptable limits. And it knows which foreign substances are harmless, such as chicken, vegetables, or pollen, for example, and which are harmful, such as toxins, viruses, and parasites.

But when the immune system is compromised, it may fail in a number of ways. For example, if it doesn't recognize a threat, it will admit into the body infectious organisms or toxins. If it mistakes friendly substances, such as foods or pollens, for harmful ones, it will produce antibodies against them and create conditions such as allergies. If it doesn't control cell reproduction properly, then cancer—a form of cell division gone out of control—results. Finally, if a stressor that does get past the immune system causes damage deep within tissue or bone, the immune system may attack that tissue or bone. Autoimmune diseases

Inflammation Is a Good Sign

When an area becomes inflamed, it means that blood flow to that spot has increased. The greater flow of blood brings important immune cells that keep the area clean and safe so it can heal. Injuries and infections need this support from the immune system so the living terrain can return to homeostasis. In holistic thinking, acute inflammation is a part of the healing process; although it may be gently soothed, it must not be suppressed. *Chronic* inflammation, on the other hand, reveals a weak living terrain or the presence of an inappropriate stressor, or both. In either case, the holistic approach supports the living terrain and takes steps to reduce the problem stress.

such as type 1 diabetes, rheumatoid arthritis, and lupus may result. (Chapter 8 covers allergies, cancer, and autoimmune conditions and their relation to stress in more depth.)

Just like the stress response system, the immune system runs by the grace of an animal's available energy and draws upon it as needed. Once again, a pet's need to rest and recover from stress is paramount to her well-being. Both while your dog or cat is fighting an infection such as a virus and after she has overcome it, she will feel tired and want to rest from her normal activities. She needs that rest. The amount of energy she can recover will affect her immune system's ability to do its job.

Just as they do for the living terrain in general, positive stress strengthens the immune system and negative stress undermines it.

STRESS AND THE IMMUNE SYSTEM

A client named Candy brought in a Rottweiler of unknown history, whom she had adopted through a rescue organization. Rory was not a healthy specimen, which is typical of many animals who have been abandoned and spent time in crowded shelters. He had major skin problems, had chronic gastrointestinal disturbances, and was aggressive

How to Measure a Pet's Immunity

Your veterinarian can help you determine your companion's susceptibility to specific viruses. With a simple blood test, you can obtain an antibody *titer* for canine distemper virus, parvovirus, feline panleukopenia, and many others. A titer measures the antibody level a pet has built up against a virus. If her immunity is low, the holistic approach provides many ways to help strengthen it. (For more on titering, see page 112.)

and hard to handle. All these issues are examples of problems that prolonged stress can create if not recognized and addressed.

To help Rory overcome his physical ailments, I recommended a diet based on unprocessed foods. I also advised Candy to work directly with an animal behaviorist to help Rory adjust to his new life in a gentler world than the one he may have known before.

After just a few weeks on the unprocessed diet, Rory's skin and digestive tract showed major improvement—the difference was like night and day. Over the next few years, Rory gradually calmed down and became very good with Candy, who was deeply committed to him. Observing Rory when he came to the clinic, I suspect that he had an issue with men because he was much more at ease with the female staff. If a dog has been abused this can be difficult to overcome, but it's something we can know about and manage. Thanks to Candy's dedication and tireless work with his behavioral issues, Rory's situation became manageable rather than impossible, giving him the benefit of a less stressful and more enjoyable life.

We don't yet understand all the ways in which stress influences the immune system and produces physical problems such as the skin and digestive issues that Rory experienced. But here's an example of how it can work. When the immune system faces an acute stressor, it increases the number of white blood cells available. Because these play a crucial role in fighting off invaders, a white blood cell population boom will help vanquish a threat.

But when stress becomes chronic and an animal doesn't recover over time, her white blood cell count *drops*. Because leukocytes protect against infections, toxins, and cancer, she must produce enough of them or she will become vulnerable to these threats.

Overall, both the stress response system and the immune system depend on an abundant supply of energy, which, in turn, they burn up as they carry out their functions in keeping our pets alive. Each system does best if the body's living terrain is in good shape to begin with, and they don't do so well if it isn't. Negative stress, whether chronic or acute, makes both the stress response system and the immune system less effective in protecting our dogs and cats. On the other hand, recent research has shown that reducing negative stress has the effect of *boosting* the immune response.[5] In sum, reducing stress not only eliminates the cause of a dog or cat's unwellness or illness, but also, through boosting the immune system, it improves her state of wellness.

Whereas Rory the Rottweiler's skin and digestive problems came from both poor diet and emotional stress, Cory the terrier's rash showed how emotional stress alone may lead to a physical health problem. But whether stress is physical, emotional, or mental in origin, it affects every aspect of our pets' health. We've seen that positive stress boosts the immune system and general wellness, while negative stress depletes energy, damages tissues, and pushes the body until it is unable to elliminate cellular by-products that can damage it. Too much negative stress can make a cat or dog vulnerable to viruses, bacteria, toxins, or parasites; weaken organs and vital systems; or turn her body against itself through autoimmune disease or cancer. Stress can cause an almost infinite range of trouble for a pet and only a health care perspective that's broad, inclusive, and flexible can address the possibilities. By taking a holistic approach and learning how to manage our pets' stress, we can make an enormous difference to their well-being and happiness.

With the philosophy of the new holistic way and the science of stress solidly behind us, we're ready to look at the kinds of stress a pet may experience. The next chapter will show you how to protect your dog or cat from negative stress.

ENDNOTES

1. George P. Chrousos et al, eds., "Stress: Basic Mechanisms and Clinical Implications," *Annals of the New York Academy of Sciences* 71 (1995). Constantine A. Stratakis and George P. Chrousos, "Neuroendocrinology and Pathophysiology of the Stress System," *Annals of the New York Academy of Sciences* 71 (1995): 1–18.
2. Jacqueline Parkin and Bryony Cohen, "An Overview of the Immune System," *The Lancet* 357, no. 9270 (2001): 1777–89.
3. The order of a dog's responses has been prioritized by dog behavior expert Silvia Jay. (For more, see sidebar "How Dogs Respond to New Situations" in this chapter.)
4. When the body is under stress, cells produce potentially harmful by-products such as free radicals and lactic acid. This process is the same in dogs, cats, and humans.
5. Richard J. Davidson et al, "Alternatives in Brain and Immune function Produced by Mindfulness Meditation," *Psychosomatic Medicine* 65 (2003): 564–70.

PART TWO

Managing Stress

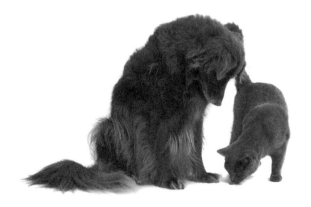

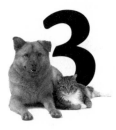

Tuning into Your Pet's Needs

When a German shorthaired pointer named Flyball suddenly began to have seizures, her veterinarian considered a possible brain tumor and similar causes. But Jeannine, her person, was reluctant to let Flyball have any invasive tests or treatments unless it was necessary, and she wasn't convinced that it was. She wanted to take some time to think about whether there might be a simpler explanation for Flyball's condition. Having recently read that chemicals in household products could cause a variety of physical problems, she wondered whether the dog could have been poisoned by a detergent or other product she used to clean the house. Jeannine was a collector of porcelain bowls that she cleaned with hydrochloric acid, and she had recently given one of her favorites to Flyball as a water dish. Jeannine removed the bowl from Flyball and the dog's seizures stopped soon afterward—thereby saving her from the added stress of medical intervention.

Most of the time, you're the first to know when your pet has a problem. After all, you eat, sleep, groom yourselves, rest, and play in each other's space. You watch each other, communicate through word and gesture, and breathe the same air. This is why you—more than your veterinarian or anyone else—carry the lion's share of responsibility when it comes to keeping your cat or dog as well and happy as possible. You're in the best position to figure out what's causing the stress that's causing your pet's problems. You're also the one who can fix them, or even—as Jeannine did at first—create them. Being responsible for your pet's wellness doesn't mean you should be able to control *everything*—no one can. But it *does* mean that you have more power than you may realize to help keep her well.

The best way to support your pet's present and future wellness is through stress prevention. To do this, you need to tune into the kinds of stress that may affect your pet and then stress-proof the ways you look after her daily needs. This chapter and the next will show you how.

Become Your Pet's Stress Monitor

Flyball's story reveals that no matter how caring we are, we may not immediately realize that something in the environment we share with our pets is causing them negative stress.

We humans may be slow on the uptake for two reasons. First, because we take so many cues from human culture instead of Nature, practices that are out of balance with the natural world may come to seem natural to us. For instance, Jeannine wanted to get rid of potentially dangerous bacteria and she accepted the cultural wisdom that the best way to do this is by using harsh industrial chemicals. Although her concern was valid, she did not consider the possible effects of such chemicals on her dog. What's more, our pets may enjoy many of our practices along with us. What dog or cat, given the chance, wouldn't gladly snooze on a comfy new foam-filled sofa even if it gives off toxic gases? But even the most adaptable animals experience negative stress when they are exposed to environmental conditions that are not appropriate for them, and this causes them to lose wellness.

Second, we can be slow to recognize stressors that affect our dogs and cats because our pets' sensory organs are much more highly developed than ours. We may not detect factors that are hard on them. But by paying attention to the sensory abilities that we do have, we can strengthen them.

You can hone your ability to notice when something clashes with your pet's needs by becoming your pet's *stress monitor*. You won't need to take notes or keep journals. All you need to do is become more attuned to your pet by using your common senses—all six of them.

We share with our pets the ability to sense the world around us through smelling, hearing, seeing, tasting, and feeling. When we lose one of these abilities, we sense the environment through the rest. Individuals who can't use all five physical senses develop the remaining ones more strongly.

However, the five physical senses don't pick up all stressors. Radiation is an example of a stressor we don't normally feel. So it's helpful that humans, cats, and dogs also share an ability to sense when someone else isn't feeling well. Whether we think of it as an instinct felt more in the body or an intuition more consciously known, most of us have it to some degree. For example, as you'll see in Chapter 6, even though his laboratory tests were clear, Jennifer was convinced that her Shetland sheepdog, Jesse, suffered from some kind of negative stress, and it turned out she was right. Chances are you've had similar experiences.

To attune your senses to what your pet may experience, first ask yourself what *you're* experiencing. Then think about how it might affect a sensitive dog or cat. Check out your pet. Does she seem restless or uncomfortable—even subtly so? She may be trying to tell you that the music is too loud for her ears or that the air freshener or other perfumed product hurts her delicate olfactory receptors. Or she may be trying to tolerate the stress by panting in a corner or sleeping. **Animals must accept the choices we make for them, so it's our responsibility to take their highly refined senses into account.**

You may feel that I am going overboard about very small issues. That's understandable, because I'm asking you to consider changing some of your habits, and habits can be hard to change. Let me assure you that I am not trying to tell you how to live. Instead, I am asking you to become aware of how your lifestyle choices may expose your dog or cat to various sources of stress. If you decide to change some of these choices, I believe that your pet's chances of achieving a greater state of wellness will increase, as may your own. You don't have to change everything, but once you make one change, you may find it will become easier to make others. Soon enough, you will begin to experience these changes as new habits that you follow without thinking. Remember: every bit helps. Even a simple act, such as making sure your pet has a quiet room or corner to retreat to while you're vacuuming, will make a difference.

USE ALL YOUR SENSES

By sharpening your senses, you'll soon find yourself noticing more. In fact, you may notice that your pet was already aware of the very thing you just picked up on.

Scent. Ask yourself, "What do I smell?" You can be sure that you don't smell as many things or as well as your dog or cat does. It never ceases to amaze me, when I'm opening a package of cheese, how the cats materialize in the kitchen from distant places as though they had just beamed in from a spaceship.

Dogs and cats sniff the air to find out what's going on in their world just the way people listen to the news. But because we humans don't rely on smell as much as we do on our other senses, we may not be sensitive to how our sealed-off modern houses and cars prevent our pets from receiving enough olfactory news to keep them in touch with their world. Cutting dogs and cats off from smells—and sounds—deprives them of sensory stimulation, and thereby contributes to boredom, one of the most serious stressors pets face today.

Make sure your dog or cat has regular access to fresh air to monitor. Leave the house or car window open a crack. Also, make sure that your pet's olfactory receptors are not overwhelmed or irritated by artificial scents such as those found in room sprays, plug-ins, perfumes, and cleaning products, or by concentrated natural scents such as those found in some herbal flea collars or aromatherapy oils. Remember that your dog or cat will not escape the strong-smelling scent of the collar fastened right under her nose any more than we could escape the assault of sound if someone strapped headphones to our ears and turned up the volume.

Hearing. "What do I hear?" We humans share with our pets a reliance on sound to connect to the world around us. However, dogs and cats hear sounds at higher and lower frequencies and over greater distances than humans do.[1] Sounds that are comfortable to our ears, such as music from our stereos, children playing, or the background hum of a refrigerator, may be amplified in our pets' ears, possibly at times to a stressful degree. They may also include pitches that we don't hear but they do—painfully—such as the high-pitched squeal of a vacuum cleaner.

Because we have chosen to share our lives and homes with dogs and cats, we should be willing to minimize for them the stressful effects of living in our sound-filled world. We can play loud music when our pets are not around. We can close the windows until the lawn mower outside stops. Clients have sometimes complained to me that a dog or cat becomes reclusive when people arrive. Through questioning them, I've often found out that, rather than being shy, their pet is escaping from a noisy crowd of people. Some pets find even a small, relatively quiet gathering overwhelming. The best thing you can do in these situations is provide your pet with a comfortable retreat and not insist that she join the crowd.

Sight. "What do I see?" Generally speaking, because dogs and cats can rely on their strong senses of sound and smell, they do not have to rely as much as most humans do on their sense of vision. In fact, dogs, and especially cats who are nocturnal, have evolved in a natural world in which darkness offers them some advantages. In the natural world, canines and felines are free to shift as they need to between relative light and darkness. They crawl into their dens to sleep in darkness and safety. They move about after evening falls or go out during the day. In other words, they are not subjected to lighting that's exactly the same for prolonged periods of time. Rather, it constantly changes. Even species that have lived with people for generations have not been exposed to steady artificial light until recently when we developed the technology to achieve it. While artificial lighting allows us to extend our vision into the darkness, both the intensity and the ubiquity of artificial lights may be stressful for our pets—not to mention ourselves. Does your pet spend most of the day in a house that's dimly lit, or in a room with a relentless bright light? To help with this, you can vary artificial light and adjust curtains to control natural light and make sure that there are places in the house where your pet can retreat into darkness or avoid overly focused lighting, such as track lights and some of the new energy-saving fluorescents that can be extremely intense.

Taste. "What do I taste?" Imagine if all you ever ate was dry breakfast cereal. You would soon find it boring, not to mention lacking the range of nutrients you need for proper nourishment. Just like us, our dogs and cats need a diet that allows them to experience a variety of tastes while providing them with the right balance of carbohydrates, fats, protein, and fiber to support good health.

Not all dogs or cats prefer the same tastes and textures, so pay attention to your pet's food preferences: give her what she likes and don't push her to eat what she dislikes. Also allow for her tastes to change over time, just as yours do. If you feed your pet treats from your table, be aware that extreme flavors may be uncomfortable or even painful for her. For example, never offer an unsuspecting animal very spicy food or hot sauce. Many pets don't like vinegar, lemon, or brine, and giving them food with these ingredients mixed in may add stress to the eating experience, which should be pleasurable. (See The Stress-Busters Diet for Dogs and Cats in the Appendix.)

Touch. "What does this feel like?" Hot or cold, smooth or rough, soft or hard—a dog or cat's sense of touch will sometimes match yours, but other times it won't. For example, a cat may enjoy lying near a hot radiator longer than most humans would. And a northern breed of dog may enjoy cooling his jets for a while in a snowbank and even prefer living outdoors; being indoors may stress him out because it is too warm for him. On the other hand, just because some dogs love the snow doesn't mean that they *should* be left out in it all day. Balance is the key. What does *your* pet need?

We humans have learned to wait for hot food to cool to a safe and comfortable temperature. But the average dog will try to wolf down a hot treat and will be surprised and possibly burned in the process. So stick your fingertip into the center of a cooked treat to ensure that it's near to room temperature—don't trust your mouth; it'll tell you that the morsel is safe for *you* long before it's safe for your dog or cat.

Most pets love cushy, comfy places to sleep. But in hot weather they can become too warm, so they must be free to sleep in a different place if they need to. And while arthritic dogs, in particular, appreciate a nice, spongy bed to protect their bones, most dogs and cats don't mind sleeping some of the time on a hard floor—something most humans would rather *not* do. Your own tactile sense will not always be the best guide to what your dog or cat finds comfortable. Instead, observe what your individual pet prefers and find out what you can about her breed, such as their geographic origin, the jobs they were given to do, and the physical characteristics that have been bred into them. This knowledge will give you important clues to the kind of physical environment that may best suit her needs.

Instinct and intuition. "Do things seem as they should?" If not—if your pet seems unusually quiet, anxious, or wound up—take notice. He may be bothered by an environmental stressor from which he can't escape, or he may be unwell or ill. By acknowledging what you sense and considering the possibilities, you'll either realize that you had no need to be concerned, or you'll get a clue as to what might be causing your pet's problem. At the very least, you may notice stressors you might otherwise have missed.

Using your six senses to monitor stress that could affect your pet will help you come as close as a human can to experiencing his situation as *he* experiences them. But if you feel as though trying to manage it seems like sailing in an ocean of endless possibilities, you don't have to feel overwhelmed. The next step will provide you with goals to guide you as you go along.

Three Important Conditions for Pet Wellness

Even with our senses sharpened and the best of intentions, we can't free our pet's world of negative stress completely. What we can do, realistically, is create the best conditions for managing her stress. I believe that through every stage of her life three conditions are especially important for doing this and that without them her optimal wellness will not be achieved, maintained, or restored. With a little love and imagination, these three conditions are not hard to meet.

Your pet needs to be well enough to respond positively to stress. Normally, a cat or dog will respond well to stress if he has clear, vital energy and a healthy living terrain. But if a pet is already unwell or ill, he will have trouble returning to balance even if he can rest when he's tired or find shelter when he's cold.

Angus and Mindy, the dog and cat discussed in Chapter 2, bounced back beautifully from their encounters with stress because they started out with enough wellness to do so. But what might have happened if they hadn't been well enough to meet their challenges?

For example, what if Angus had a heart condition? If he played too long and hard he could put his heart into crisis and would not be able to recover on his own. Or what if Mindy had a chronic and debilitating illness such as feline leukemia? In her rundown state, she might not have the vitality to recover quickly if exposed to cold temperatures.

Angus and Mindy show us that for a pet to respond positively to stress, his or her living terrain must have enough energy and physical integrity to be able to return to homeostasis. Unwell or ill pets will end up losing wellness when they encounter negative stress.

The environment should provide your pet with appropriate stress. Healthy pets will respond positively to stress as long as it's appropriate. In fact, to thrive pets *need* appropriate stress, and in caring for our pets we must be careful not to overly protect them from stressors that would be of benefit to them. Again, balance is the key.

But some stressors are inappropriate regardless of the health of the pet. When sources of stress are out of synchronicity with a dog or cat's living terrain, even the most resilient dog or cat will have trouble dealing with them. Environmental stressors such as pesticides and cigarette smoke are examples.

Consider once again Angus and Mindy. They were exposed to stress but recovered homeostasis for two reasons: they had enough wellness to begin with, and the stressors they faced—reasonable exercise and limited exposure to extreme weather—are appropriate for most dogs and cats. But if the stressors had not been appropriate, their story would have unfolded differently.

Imagine that Angus's person Dave leaves him out in the yard after they come home from the park, instead of taking him inside. Angus longs to stretch out under the maple tree and lie low until he's recovered his balance from his afternoon of fun and games. But the neighborhood kids come over and want to play with him. Angus is a mixed breed with a little herding dog in him. It's his nature to work or play for as long as he is asked, so he responds to the children's enthusiasm and abandons his desire to rest. But in spite of his herding ancestry, Angus is a companion dog who doesn't have the athletic level of fitness that he would have if he lived a working life. So after trying to play with the kids for awhile he flops down, exhausted, panting hard and unable or unwilling to get up. His environment has provided him with stress that is inappropriate for him, even though he was generally well to begin with.

Or imagine that the temperature in Mindy's region drops abnormally low, much colder than she would typically cope with. Mindy might succumb so quickly that she couldn't make it to shelter, and could even die from exposure. Even though, like Angus, Mindy is a well pet, her environment provides stress that is too extreme for her.

Even the healthiest pets may experience inappropriate stressors that cause them to become unwell, ill, or even die. Examples may include contaminated food, air, or water; unusual temperature, humidity, or dryness; or extreme emotional and psychological disruption. (See the Eight Realms of Stress beginning on page 71.)

Your pet needs to have opportunities to help herself or have your protection as a substitute. When under stress, a pet must be able to improve her own situation. She must have opportunities either to escape from stress or to overcome it, or she will require your help to do so.

Healthy animals always try to help themselves. A dog will seek water if he's thirsty or find a place to rest if he's tired, and a cat will run up a tree to escape a dog or will climb into a warm shelter if she's cold. But in our complicated world, pets often find themselves challenged by stressors that they're not well suited to handle. That's when they need our help.

If Angus has the option, he'll probably follow Dave into the house and stretch out in a quiet corner. Or he'll let himself in if he has a doggy door. If the yard offers some shelter, he might wriggle into the cool dirt under the porch or go into his doghouse. But he still needs a fence secure enough to keep others from invading his space. All of these are options that Angus can only have available if Dave provides them.

Mindy needs her people to watch for her to let her in or provide her with a cat door to let herself in. Otherwise, she will be stuck outside in the cold for too long.

Notice what your pet can do for herself and what she needs your help to do. The more you can tune into her needs, the more you'll see ways to reduce her negative stress—whether it's physical, emotional, or environmental—and increase her positive stress.

No matter how much you may want to, you won't be able to fix everything in your pet's environment. But it will help to know the kinds of stressors to watch out for. I categorize them into eight realms of stress.

The Eight Realms of Stress

As I explained in Chapter 2, stress involves much more than being emotionally upset or under pressure. The general descriptions below will introduce you to the eight realms of stress. They're not meant to be exhaustive, but to provide a sense of what each realm involves. Once you get the gist of them, they will help you think broadly and constructively about ways to support your pet's well-being. You can use them to identify aspects of your lifestyle that may not support your pet's wellness and find ways to make them more harmonious with both your needs and hers.

GENETIC STRESS

A pet's first relationship with stress starts before conception and continues while she's in the womb and in the earliest days after she is born. I knew a pair of pups from the same litter who clearly illustrated this. Their story begins with their parents.

A healthy male German shepherd mix who had a stable temperament was bred to a female of a similar mix who was flighty and sensitive and had a history of skin problems. While the female was pregnant, her people moved with her into a new environment where another dog lived with whom she didn't get along. Due to the situation, the pregnant mother was left outside all the time when she had previously lived indoors. Plus, her people were struggling with marital tensions, so she went through her pregnancy under a great deal of stress.

Eventually, she gave birth to two pups. The male pup displayed all the characteristics of his dad—calm, well balanced, and physically robust. But the female, following after her mother, had a skittish and fearful nature and by one year of age she suffered from major skin problems, revealing a severe imbalance in her immune system. The genetic and neonatal stress that had affected this pup was very challenging to overcome. Even though I started working with her while she was young, I sometimes felt as though I was at my wit's end trying to help her get better.

It's difficult to know how much of these puppies' physical and emotional makeup resulted from their genetic inheritance versus the stress they experienced in utero. My theory is that the male inherited his more balanced genetic structure from his dad and consequently, while the puppies were developing in the womb, he was better equipped to resist the effects of their mother's stress. By contrast, the female inherited her less resilient genetic structure from her mom and was therefore more vulnerable to her mother's stress. The mother's suffering caused great stress in turn to the female pup's developing immune system, and this manifested in the health problems that plagued her from a tender age.

Dogs and cats, like humans, inherit from their ancestors genetic characteristics that predispose them to thrive in particular climates, express some abilities more than others, and establish certain kinds of social relationships. In current scientific thinking, genetic predispositions are not a permanent part of a species' makeup. Rather, they represent ways that a given species, line of ancestors, or specific ancestor adapted to stressors in the environment. Genetic stress occurs when your pet's inherited predisposition hinders, rather than supports, her ability to respond successfully to her environment. Climates, activities, and social arrangements that differ a lot from those her ancestors knew may cause her varying degrees of negative stress.[2]

Human interference may also cause genetic stress. For example, breeding dogs or cats to enhance some characteristics and eliminate others may lead to health problems such as overcrowded teeth, underbites, or overbites in pets whose jaw structures have become flattened to match a breed standard. As well, inappropriate training or lifestyle pressures, wrong diet, immunization, drugs, pollution, and being forced to live in highly unnatural environments may expose pets to challenges incompatible with their inherited predispositions.

All pets probably have some form of genetic stress. Although we can't change their genetic makeup, we can improve the way they respond when faced with challenges that are incompatible with their inheritance. By learning as much as you can about your pet's background, including her particular line of ancestors or her breed, you'll be better able to understand how to support her.

NEONATAL (NEWBORN) STRESS

Your pet will be affected throughout her life by conditions her mother experienced while she was in the womb, as well as in the earliest days after she was born. While puppies or kittens grow in utero, the negative stress their mother experiences is transmitted to them. Inappropriate diet, drugs and other artificial chemicals, and physical or emotional suffering cause changes in her hormones, tissues, and biological systems, and these changes affect her young. Toxins also pass to the litter directly. The litter and its descendants may express this stress through physical and emotional problems; in other words, neonatal stress may become genetic stress. For example, if a pregnant animal suffers emotional abuse or neglect, this can produce in her offspring behavior imbalances such as being overly fearful or aggressive, which are then passed on to subsequent generations.[3]

What puppies and kittens experience in the first days after birth also profoundly affects them. If they are deprived of their mother's nurturing, inoculated during their first two weeks, given drugs, or exposed to toxic chemicals, their future well-being will be significantly compromised. For example, a newborn who receives antibiotics will possibly end up with lifelong digestive problems and a weakened immune system, predisposing him to permanent health problems. Dogs born in puppy mills provide a dramatic example of the destructive effects of neonatal stress. These unfortunate individuals typically are plagued by significant health and behavior problems all their lives. Anything you can learn about the neonatal stress your pet may have experienced will help you support him better.

DYSBIOTIC STRESS

A client brought in a young German shepherd who had chronic diarrhea and foul-smelling skin. The cause of the trouble was a mystery; the dog's stool analysis had always been normal and contained no parasites or other clues. Gary told me that he was very tired of the situation and he felt almost ready to euthanize the dog. But instead, he brought King to me.

When taking his history, I learned that King had been treated with many bouts of antibiotics to relieve his diarrhea. When this failed, he'd been referred to a specialist to have his bowel biopsied for a definitive diagnosis. But because this would be a costly procedure and he didn't

Respect the Integrity of Your Pet's Body

Don't de-claw your cat, crop your dog's ears, or dock his tail. These practices are abnormal and unnatural. They are done for cosmetic purposes and do not provide health benefits in spite of arguments to the contrary that their advocates may put forward. Usually done at a tender age, they are inhumane and cause the animal distress. They also can produce negative stress for the animal later in life as he lives with their effects. In both respects, it's even harder on pets when these practices are carried out when they are adults. Cats are meant to have claws. Dogs are meant to have tails, and dog breeds that have specialized in various activities have developed different natural ear shapes accordingly. Let them be.

want to put the dog through that kind of stress, Gary decided against it. Subsequently, King had been placed on prescription diets—he had been through about ten different so-called hypoallergenic processed foods—but still, no dice.

I quickly concluded that King was suffering from dysbiotic stress and I told Gary I thought he could make a miraculous improvement with a few simple changes. I customized a raw diet for the dog and recommended an herbal gastrointestinal soothant plus probiotics to rebalance his digestive flora. In fact, I felt confident that King would respond if all we did was shift him to an unprocessed diet with no additional supports. Gary put all the measures in place, however, and in a matter of days King recovered almost completely.

Feeling greatly encouraged, Gary agreed to bring King back for auricular medicine assessment. This subtle form of diagnosis would guide us in fine-tuning the dog's diet along with digestive and other supports to help his body recover from its long ordeal. (See Chapter 6 for more on bioenergetic assessment, beginning on page 145.)

Why could this dog handle raw food when he could not handle processed food? I can't explain it. I only know that I've seen the same thing happen for years and years in my practice.

Dogs and cats' bodies need to contain the right balance of bacteria and other organisms to function properly. These flora are crucial to effective digestion and a strong immune system. Skin, too, relies upon friendly bacteria to help it perform its functions. When a pet's flora are out of balance, the pet experiences dysbiotic stress.[4]

Dysbiotic stress means that the living terrain contains too many unfriendly organisms and not enough friendly ones. It plays an important role in systemic problems, including inflammatory bowel disease, allergies, and more. For example, it can result in an overpopulation of yeast, which encourages both ear infections and digestive upsets. Temporary dysbiotic stress can be caused by eating or drinking inappropriate or contaminated foods or liquids, infectious diseases, and antibiotics. When used repeatedly, antibiotics cause chronic dysbiotic stress, which eventually leads to other health breakdowns. (See Iatrogenic Stress on page 81.) Eating an appropriate diet, avoiding antibiotics, and the therapeutic use of probiotics (friendly bacteria) will help correct the biotic balance.

DIETARY STRESS

Dietary stress, the result of an unsuitable diet, causes wellness to deteriorate. A proper diet should nourish cells and tissues, increase energy, and provide sensory satisfaction. It must be correctly balanced for the species and breed, and adjusted for individual allergies or sensitivities. It should not include nonfood and potentially toxic additives, such as fillers, cosmetic enhancers, industrial preservatives, or drugs. When a pet's diet doesn't meet these criteria her wellness will suffer, and her living terrain will lose vitality and the ability to bounce back when other stressors challenge her.[5] (See Fulleh's story in Chapter 4, beginning on page 105.)

Leave Inner Ear Hairs and Anal Glands Alone

Don't invade your pet's living terrain without true medical need. For example:

Don't pull hair out of your dog's ears. The hair is a natural cleansing device, so you never need to put cleaning agents of any kind into her ears. If her ears are dysbiotic and have become infected this normally signals an underlying systemic problem that needs to be addressed through dietary adjustments and supportive therapies.

Don't let anyone squeeze your pet's anal glands without medical justification. These glands are part of an olfactory recognition system that dogs use to identify each other. They express a substance on stools when the animal has a bowel movement. Emptying them is a horrible experience for the animal and serves no purpose since the glands fill up again and return to their natural state. Infection or blockage is a sign of rectal dysbiosis that requires holistic support. For regular maintenance, a balanced, unprocessed diet based on meat and bones will produce stools of the ideal, bulky consistency that will keep a dog's anal glands expressing themselves as they should.

Since the mid-twentieth century, dogs and cats' diets have become less suited to their living terrains, particularly in relation to the increased use of processed pet foods.[6] Pets display diet-related health problems that range from subtle unwellness to all manner of illnesses. Unwellness has become so much the norm among pets that it's safe to say many people have never seen or don't know what a truly well dog or cat should look like. In the dog park, on the streets, and in private homes, animals who lack luster in their coats, eyes, and energy levels are taken to be well. It's now so common for dogs and cats to become seriously *ill* during their lifetimes that many pet lovers appear to have resigned themselves to the notion that this comes with the territory of having a pet. This situation is tragic. Evidence has shown that most illnesses that afflict pets today were rarely, if ever, seen before we began feeding dogs and cats processed foods. (See Chapter 4 for more on stress and diet, and The Stress-Busters Diet for Dogs and Cats in the Appendix.)

EMOTIONAL STRESS

When Millie, a tortoiseshell cat, came into the clinic with a swollen lip, we also found telltale acne on her chin. These common lesions, called eosinophilic granulomatosis, often progress to the animal's lips and ulcerate, sometimes badly. Caused by latent viruses, they flare up when the cat is under emotional stress. Stress suppresses the immune system and the viruses take advantage of this. Chin acne and lip ulcers are surefire indicators of a cat's stress level.

These viruses don't respond to antibiotics even though the latter are often used to treat them. However, because the acne and ulcers are inflammatory reactions, steroids can suppress them. But steroids also lower the body's immune response, which it needs to fight the viruses. To deal with this affliction properly, we must look at what is going on in the patient's life.

As I talked with Millie's guardian, Debbie, I learned that she had taken in her parents' dog while they had gone down south for the winter. The dog was not cat-aggressive, but he was young and rambunctious, which made Millie nervous. Together, we came up with a way to relieve Millie's stress. Debbie realized she could make one of the cat's favorite rooms off-limits to the dog so Millie could count on it as a safe retreat, and I added some flower remedies to the plan.

A short time after this, Millie's lip began to clear up. By modifying the source of her emotional stress, her virus lost its foothold and returned to its latent state.

Because pets often seem to adapt so well to their circumstances, we may not always recognize the emotional stress in their lives. But when circumstances either don't meet a pet's emotional needs or clash with them, he will experience emotional stress. Emotional stress sets off

Help Your Pet Cope with *Your* Emotional Stress

Dogs and cats are caring, sensitive creatures who become highly attuned to the ones they love. They tend to take care of *our* emotional needs, so when we are emotionally stressed they will be affected. For example, tension between family members can stress pets severely. So can moving, as well as people or animals joining the family or leaving it.

When you go through your own tough emotional times, you can help your pet cope. Reassure her that her place is with you and that your love for her won't change. Play with her or go for a walk with her: you may soon find yourself shifting out of your worries, and both of you will benefit. Flower remedies (see page 166) can gently support an animal who suffers from emotional stress. Finally, if a beloved person or animal dies or leaves, your pet may grieve. *Don't confuse grief with negative stress.* In animals, as with people, grief must be compassionately received. Negative stress sets in when grief is *not* given the space and time it needs.

a cascade of cellular and hormonal reactions. When extreme or prolonged, stress expresses itself through physical or behavioral problems such as skin reactions, fear-aggression, withdrawal, and more. And it makes pets more susceptible to many forms of illness.[7]

Abuse and neglect are obvious causes of not only physical but also emotional stress. Other sources are more subtle. For example, because a dog's sense of security derives from knowing his place in a pack or family, he becomes anxious and insecure when his position isn't clear. A cat can be very stressed out by the presence of another cat she dislikes. Boredom and loneliness are profound sources of emotional stress for both species. Dogs and cats should never spend long hours trapped in isolation; this causes anguish for dogs even more than for cats, and its effect on both animals' long-term health, must not be underestimated.

By being aware of the situations that cause pets emotional stress, we can find ways to alleviate them.

ENVIRONMENTAL STRESS

Years ago I took my car into a body shop for repair. While there, I met Dale the Doberman, who guarded the place and lived in the shop where the work was done. When the shop's owner-mechanic said that Dale wasn't a healthy dog, I mentioned that I was a veterinarian and said, "Bring him over to my clinic and we'll see what's going on."

When Dale came for his appointment, I learned that he had a poor appetite and chronic digestive problems. He also scratched himself a lot and had flaking skin and a poor coat. Yet he had a zest for life and carried out with vigor his role of guarding the shop.

Blood and urine tests told us that Dale had liver and kidney problems and signs of multiple degenerative conditions. We sent some of his hair away for analysis and found out from this that he had toxic levels of lead, aluminum, arsenic, and other serious mineral abnormalities.

Dale's body was under terrific environmental stress from fighting a chemical overload. It wasn't hard to figure out why; he lived in less than ideal cleanliness and was constantly exposed to many minerals, chemicals, and heavy metals involved with car body repair. The answer for Dale would be to improve his diet and change his environment.

The mechanic set Dale up to live outside the shop and put him on a more wholesome diet. With these changes, the dog's body mass improved—he digested better and gained weight, and his coat grew in thicker and healthier. If I'd seen his case today, I'd have other supportive therapies at my disposal—I would use homeopathic drainage remedies to detoxify his kidneys and liver and his body in general. I'd also add antioxidants and vitamin and mineral supplements. But even without these additional supports, I was delighted with how much he improved. I believe we saved his life, because I think he would have died if left in the circumstances in which I first saw him.

Just as Dale did, pets experience environmental stress when pollutants and toxins challenge their living terrain. Pollutants and toxins may be biological, such as bacteria in decaying meats; chemical, such as phthalates used to soften vinyl plastics and melamine added to the food supply; or energetic, such as radiation leaking from toxic waste sites and natural radon from the bedrock beneath the home. Household cleaners can be major sources of environmental stressors. If you use air fresheners or room deodorizers, think about the chemical load your pet may breathe in or lick off his feet and fur after walking and lying on sprayed surfaces. Very little legislation exists to ensure that household products are safe for pets.[8]

Environmental stressors may be present in almost anything your pet eats, drinks, breathes, and walks, plays, bathes, and lies in or on, including water; food, and treats; kitty litter; toys; collars, muzzles, and harnesses; shampoos and conditioners; flea, tick, and heartworm products; and pharmaceutical drugs. Although they're often included as standard ingredients in mass-produced products, they also show up in some products that claim to be natural. Learn to read labels carefully. None of us can completely avoid environmental stressors, but by making careful choices we can cut back on how much we expose our pets to them.

IATROGENIC STRESS

A female Yorkshire terrier named Tara was presented to an emergency clinic for evaluation of progressive neurological abnormalities. Her first signs had appeared about six weeks before, just hours after she had received her second injection of a particular multivalent vaccine. At first she had weakness in her hind limbs, which seemed to improve over a month's time. But then she flew with her people to Spain, and

More Toxins in Pets Than in People

Animals live closer to the ground than we do. When they come across something they want to investigate, they sniff it, stick their faces into it, often taste it, and may even lap it up. Because they don't wear shoes, their bare paws directly contact what may be on the ground. So pets are especially vulnerable to harmful chemicals that may leach from manufactured products.

In 2008, the Environmental Working Group (EWG) of the United States checked the blood and urine of twenty dogs and thirty-seven cats for seventy chemicals commonly present in household products and furniture. They found that both species were contaminated with forty-eight of these chemicals, forty-three of them at higher levels than those typically found in people. And compared to people in national studies conducted by the Centers for Disease Control and Prevention as well as the EWG, dogs showed nearly two and a half times greater levels of stain- and grease-proof coatings (perfluorochemicals). Cats had twenty-three times more fire retardants (PBDEs) and more than five times the amount of mercury.[9]

Secondhand smoke's potential threat to your pet should also raise your hackles. The Québec Lung Association states that along with its effects on people, "Second-hand smoke also affects the health of household pets. Their fur coat traps the smoke particles which the animals then absorb when they groom themselves. Second-hand smoke may cause leukemia in cats, and increases the risk of cancer in dogs."[10]

the stress of the travel set her back. There, she began circling to the left with her head tilted to the right, had trouble seeing, and became extremely weak.

Back home again at the emergency clinic, she still circled to the left but now dragged her hind legs behind her. She did not have full vision in her right eye, and when she was turned over she panicked and twisted her back to the right. She did not know where her hind legs were, and when her head was touched she overreacted. The clinic staff knew they were dealing with a severe neurological problem and wanted to do an MRI scan, but the clients declined. Unable to carry out further diagnostics, the vets treated Tara with prednisone.

At this stage, Tara's people brought her to us. Although we could not prove it, we assumed that the vaccination had introduced toxicity into her nervous system; as researcher Jean Dodds has pointed out, severe reactions to vaccines are not uncommon.[11] We gave Tara homeopathics for the assumed vaccinosis and a neurological drainage remedy for nervous system toxicity. To try to energize her nervous system we added acupuncture, veterinary orthopedic manipulation (VOM), and a variety of hands-on therapies such as Reiki. And to support her living terrain as it attempted to heal, we improved her diet and provided nutraceutical supplements. We aimed to give her a reasonable quality of life.

Over many months, we slowly made progress reestablishing Tara's nervous function. It takes a long time to recuperate from severe neurological damage because nerve tissue replicates very slowly. But it is possible. The key is to use every means we have available and be persistent. It feels wonderful to see a dog in Tara's condition gradually regain control. Even though she may not recover completely, what matters is being able to bring the animal back to a life worth living.

Iatrogenic stress is caused by medical examination or treatment. Examples include the negative effects of drugs, vaccines, surgery, or radiation. Although methods such as these sometimes dramatically help patients, unfortunately they also tend to damage cells, tissues, organs, and hormonal balance because they work by attacking the living terrain. For example, radiation both destroys and causes cancer, and the steroid prednisone relieves symptoms of pain and discomfort but at the same time suppresses the immune system. In general, iatrogenic stress contributes significantly to the other types of stress.[12]

In contrast, by the very nature of what they do, remedies and therapies that *support* the living terrain—such as physiotherapy, acupuncture, homeopathy, and many more—don't pose the same dangers as methods that attack it. As a result, they do not typically damage cells, tissues, organs, or hormonal balance. Nevertheless, when not used appropriately these kinds of therapies may also cause undesirable results. (See pages 171–179.)

GERIATRIC STRESS

Sam, a fully housebroken beagle, suddenly began to defecate in the house. Because he was thirteen years old, Amanda and Ben, his people, wondered whether he might be losing control of his bowels or going senile and therefore becoming confused about where to relieve himself. Their assumptions were understandable because senior pets' problems are often mistaken for signs of aging.

Mainstream medicine might have prescribed drugs to control Sam's bowels or to make him less disoriented. But Amanda wasn't satisfied that these were his problems. Instead, she thought about whether changes that occured just before his behavior altered might have stressed him out. She made several observations.

First, Sam left his poop in their five-year-old daughter Noah's bedroom and playroom and nowhere else. So it was unlikely he had lost control of his bowels. But why would he choose only those rooms? Looking back, Amanda recalled that when Noah was born, Sam had switched his attachment from Ben to herself. Plus, Sam had recently become too stiff to get up onto their bed at night and so had started sleeping on the floor. They also had a new kitten who had moved into Sam's old place on their bed. It dawned on Amanda that Sam had begun to relieve himself in Noah's rooms right after he had given up sleeping on the bed and the kitten had taken his place. Maybe Sam was feeling displaced and no longer sure about where he fit into the family.

To experiment, Amanda decided to give Sam a set of steps that he could climb to get onto the bed and encourage him to use them.

This would reassure him that he had not lost his place in the family. If necessary, they would gently move the kitty over to make it clear to both animals that Sam was also entitled to sleep there.

As soon as Sam got his steps he stopped relieving himself in the house. Amanda was thrilled. "He's in all-around better spirits!" Her instincts had been right—Sam wasn't senile and he hadn't lost control of his bodily functions. Rather, aging had limited his mobility and this, combined with his probable feeling of displacement as the family added more kids and animals, had caused him emotional stress that in his case was easy to remedy.

Even though age itself does not cause stress, Sam's story illustrates that age is associated with other factors that may cause stress. For example, older pets' muscles naturally decline, so they need less exercise and protein than they once did. Too much exercise and too much protein in their senior years will cause negative stress. And the longer a pet lives, the more other kinds of stress have time to take hold. For example, older pets have had longer to build up toxins or lose wellness from inappropriate diet, environmental pollution, inadequate shelter, emotional stress, and other factors. Long-term imbalances cause tissues and systems to break down. As a result, older pets may become unwell or develop illnesses they didn't have as youngsters, such as diabetes, arthritis, heart trouble, and cancer. On the other hand, with age some cancers and other illnesses may progress more slowly.[13]

Older pets are also vulnerable to various forms of cognitive dysfunction in the same way humans are. For example, recent research confirms that cats may suffer from Alzheimer's [14] and senior dogs may be affected by canine cognitive dysfunction.[15] The symptoms of these conditions are similar in both dogs and cats, although in cats they are more subtle. They include disorientation, such as aimless wandering and failing to recognize words or people that used to be very familiar to them; changes in their relationships to people, such as no longer wanting to be petted; changes in behavior, such as sleeping more or becoming restless at night; and breaking the pattern of house training, such as urinating or defecating in their sleeping areas.

But we may often assume that aging is the default explanation for all kinds of changes in a pet's behavior, just as we may with human behavior. So, as in Sam's case, a change in a geriatric pet's behavior might *look* like senile dementia when other stressors are the cause of his trouble. For example, when senior pets have difficulty climbing or jumping they lose access to sofas, beds, and other favorite resting places they cherish. Dogs consider it a privilege to sleep near their people, at least in part because it is as a sign of their position in the group and they derive security from this. Losing access to precious places can make an aging pet anxious, especially if another pet takes it over. Don't assume that your aging pet is senile until you've thought about what else may have changed in his life and how you might be able to improve it.

Because an older pet's cells and tissues won't respond to change as quickly as those of a younger pet, your effort to support the living terrain of your older dog or cat will probably take longer to have an effect—but it *will* make a difference. It's almost never too late to detoxify and nourish your pet's living terrain and adjust her environment so she can become more well. Even in cases of terminal illness, holistic care will improve the quality of the time that a pet has left.

Now that we've looked at the kinds of stress a pet may experience, we're ready to talk about stress-proofing her daily life. Chapter 4 provides practical guidelines to help you do this.

ENDNOTES

1. Laura Hungerford, "Dog Hearing," Ask a Scientist(c), Veterinary Topics Archive, United States Department of Energy, www.newton.dep.anl.gov/askasci/vet00/vet00003.htm (accessed December 22, 2008); Rickye S. Heffner and Henry E. Heffner, "Hearing Range of the Domestic Cat," *Hearing Research* 19, no. 1 (1985): 85–8.
2. Rudolf Bijlsma and Volker Loeschcke, eds., *Environmental Stress, Adaptation, and Evolution* (Boston: Birkhåuser, 1997).
3. Christine C. Johnson et al, "Antibiotic Exposure in Early Infancy and Risk for Childhood Atopy," *The Journal of Allergy and Clinical Immunology* 115, no. 6 (June 2005): 1218–24; Alain Gagnon et al, "Obstetrical Complications Associated with Abnormal Maternal Serum Markers Analytes," *Journal of Obstetric and Gynaecology Canada* 30, no. 10 (October 2008): 918–32.
4. Eamonn M. Quigley, "Bacteria: A New Player in Gastrointestinal Motility Disorders—Infections, Bacterial Overgrowth, and Probiotics," *Gastroenterology Clinics of North America* 36, no. 3 (September 2007): 735–48; Tomasz Mach, "Clinical Usefulness of Probiotics in Inflammatory Bowel Diseases," *Journal of Physiological Pharmacology* 57, Supplement 9 (November 2006): 23–33.
5. Mohammed Hossein Noyan-Ashraf et al, "Phase 2 Protein Inducers in the Diet Promote Healthier Aging," *The Journals of Gerontology, Series A, Biological Sciences and Medical Sciences* 63, no. 11 (November 2008): 1168–76; Maxim E. Darvin et al, "One-year Study on the Variation of Carotenoid Antioxidant Substances in Living Human Skin: Influence of Dietary Supplementation and Stress Factors," *Journal of Biomedical Optics* 13, no. 4 (July-August 2008): 044028.
6. For a detailed discussion of how pets' diets have changed in the last half century and how this has affected their health, see The Stress-Busters Diet for Dogs and Cats in the Appendix.
7. Luis Vitetta et al, "Mind-body Medicine: Stress and Its Impact on Overall Health and Longevity," *Annals of the New York Academy of Sciences* 1057 (December 2005): 492–505.
8. Sattar Ansar Ahmed, "The Immune System as a Potential Target for Environmental Estrogens (Endocrine Disrupters): A New Emerging Field," *Toxicology* 150, Issues 1–3, 7 (September 2000): 191–206.
9. Olga Naidenko, Rebecca Sutton, and Jane Houlihan, "High Levels of Toxic Industrial Chemicals Contaminate Cats and Dogs," Environmental Working Group, April 2008, www.ewg.org/reports/pets (accessed April 16, 2009).

10. "Second-hand Smoke in the Environment," The Lung Association: Québec, www.pq.lung.ca/services/poumon-9/smoke-fumee/ (accessed April 16, 2009).

11. W. Jean Dodds, "Adverse Vaccine Reactions," Britfield Weimariners, www.britfeld.com/vaccination-adverse.htm (accessed December 17, 2008).

12. Sally E. Jensen et al, "Virally Mediated Cervical Cancer in the Iatrogenically Immunocompromised: Applications for Psychoneuroimmunology," *Brain, Behaviour, and Immunity* 21, no. 6 (August 2007): 758–66; Richard R. Bootzin and Elaine T. Bailey, "Understanding Placebo, Nocebo, and Iatrogenic Treatment Effects," *Journal of Clinical Psychology* 61, no. 7 (July 2005): 871–80.

13. Margot Shields and Laurent Martel, "Healthy Living Among Seniors," *Health Reports/Statistics Canada*, Canadian Centre for Health Information, Supplement 16 (2006): 7–20; Diane B. Miller and James P. O'Callaghan, "Aging, Stress and the Hippocampus," *Ageing Research Reviews* 4, no. 2 (May 2005): 123–40.

14. Danielle Gunn-Moore et al, "Cognitive Dysfunction and the Neurobiology of Ageing in Cats," *Journal of Small Animal Practice* 48 (October 2007): 546–53.

15. Jacqueline C. Neilson et al, "Prevalence of Behavioral Changes Associated with Age-related Cognitive Impairment in Dogs," *Journal of the American Veterinary Medical Association* 218, no. 11 (June 1, 2001): 1787–91.

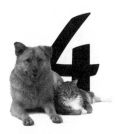

Preventing Stress in Daily Life

Prevention has always been the best guarantee for long-term wellness, and this is as true when it comes to managing our pets' stress as it is for managing our own. This chapter will help you stress-proof your pet's home life, diet, exercise, and general care. By taking steps to prevent negative stress from happening in our dogs or cats' futures, we can ensure that many health problems that they *might* have had don't develop at all.

As we saw with Flyball, the pointer whose person unwittingly exposed her to cleaning chemicals, pets can be stressed out by sources that we might not think of right away. This brings us to a key difference between pets and their wild cousins. Whereas the wilderness provides animals with opportunities to avoid negative stressors, domestic life severely restricts these choices for animals who are pets. Pets pretty well have to put up with the conditions we create for them. As a result, the most important choice you'll ever make on your pet's behalf is to pick an animal whose needs are compatible with your own. Whenever possible, the place to start your research is *before* you adopt.

What Kind of Pet Are *You* Right For?

After her husband of many years died, Cora longed for the companionship of a dog. She wanted to make her choice carefully, so before she adopted she asked me which breed of dog might fit her situation. Because Cora was tiny and lived in a small place, she'd been thinking that a small dog such as a Parson Russell terrier might work out. But Cora herself was not very active.

I told her I didn't think a terrier would work for her. They tend to be high-energy dogs and require a more intense level of activity than Cora herself kept up. A small terrier might fit her criteria for size, but not for other practical concerns.

I suggested she think about a bigger dog. Some large breeds are very calm and require less activity to satisfy their needs. Even a St. Bernard might have worked out in her case.

Cora went out and got an Irish wolfhound puppy. Although Artie grew up to be bigger than she was, they had a wonderful relationship. Artie was a great big couch potato, as Irish wolfhounds often are, and the two of them shared their small abode contentedly. In spite of his size, Cora never had any special problems handling him, and their relationship blossomed. Artie became her whole life. They were totally into each other. It was a perfect match. Even though it seemed superficially incompatible, it worked out very, very well.

Having a pet is not like owning a piece of furniture, a toy, or a gadget that can be ignored when you're not using it. An animal requires commitment, attention, relationship, time, energy, and money—as does a child—and the pet will need these from you for as long as it would take a human child to grow up. A dog may live fifteen years and a cat, twenty. This is why it's crucial to ask yourself serious questions about your lifestyle and future *before* you adopt.

Your pet will depend on you for its entire life, a span of time that may involve several major changes in your own life circumstances. So, start by honestly considering your personal needs. Then learn all you can about the needs of the animal you wish to adopt. If your needs will conflict with those of the animal, *don't adopt* that kind of pet. Choose an animal whose needs will fit with your lifestyle—unless you will allow yourself to change so that you can meet that animal's needs. Remember: *you* have the choice in this matter. The animal does not. By being honest with yourself about what you're ready for and choosing a pet accordingly, you can save your pet from a stressful future and the inevitable health problems that would bring.

For example, are you gone twelve hours a day? Do you, or will you, live in a small apartment without your own yard? In either case, *don't* get a big, frisky dog such as a German shepherd. Your situation won't meet the needs of this high-energy breed and will create a very stressful environment for him. A dog like this needs companionship and daily exercise. It simply won't work to keep him indoors in an apartment building or alone all day.

What's your life going to be like in six months or a decade from now? Will you leave for school in a year or two, or travel a lot? I often see pets who were left with the parents of a grown-up child who left the nest. The parents may not really want the pet, and though they may look after it, the love and commitment the animal needs is not always there. Might you have kids soon? Don't get a pet if you expect big life changes within the next few years. Wait until you have made those changes and can assess how a pet will fit with them.

Once you have decided that you have room in your life for a pet, you will need to choose what kind of pet you will adopt. Both dogs and cats need love and attention, but dogs need a constant level of involvement that will put a serious damper on your own freedom. Are you sure this is what you want?

After you've chosen the type of animal you want to share your life with, you need to think about its individual characteristics. The characteristics and needs of purebreds may be more predictable. For

Look after Your Pet—Look after Yourself

Samantha spent her days working at a computer, so she didn't get much exercise and wasn't in great shape. But she loved big dogs, so she adopted a Great Dane. Little did she know that her commitment to Newton's well-being would have great payoffs for her own wellness.

Because she couldn't let Newton run around the neighborhood on his own, Samantha felt obliged to provide him with daily exercise. So she walked him twice a day and tried to make each walk last a half hour or more. And rather than holding Newton back to her slow human walking pace, she let him trot when he felt like it while she casually jogged along behind him. It made her happy to see how much Newton enjoyed his walks.

Although Samantha knew that Newton benefited from these outings, she didn't at first recognize that her own wellness was improving, too. She found this out one morning when she left Newton at home so she could attend a meeting. Realizing that she had only a minute or two to catch her bus, she sprinted the two blocks to the bus stop. As she leapt onto the vehicle it occured to her that for the first time in ages she was not out of breath from a hard run. Her stamina had increased thanks to her daily jaunts with Newton. By doing what was best for her dog, Samantha had increased her own well-being.

example, Siamese cats can be reserved, whereas Maine coon cats are sociable and outgoing. But even then, individuals vary. Mixes may display tendencies of one or more breeds. Learn about the breeds that interest you, and about the health and behavior of family lines of the individual you are considering.

An animal's age and past experience counts, too. Puppies and kittens require special care and behavior from *you* while they're young. Adult animals, whether rescued or re-homed, will have issues from earlier situations that did not work out. Ask breeders, shelter staff, or previous owners about an animal's personality and preferences. Is she friendly, aggressive, or fearful? Clingy or confident? And in what kinds of situations? This way, you can better determine what *you* can handle and which of a pet's needs *you* are prepared to meet.

Begin with Preventing Boredom and Loneliness

Heidi, a miniature schnauzer, suffered from severe, relentless itching around her head and eyes. My client, Celeste, brought her to us after she'd been treated as an allergy case at another clinic. Heidi had to wear an Elizabethan collar around her head almost constantly to keep her from scratching.

Auricular medicine assessment (see page 151) helped us determine what Heidi should and should not eat, and we shifted her from processed, packaged food to fresh, unprocessed meats and vegetables. Heidi then made progress to the point where she was able to stop wearing the hated plastic cone.

Then Celeste and Heidi moved and Heidi's allergies returned in force, requiring her once more to don the dreaded cone. Celeste and I discussed what factors in the new environment might be creating stress for the dog. Because Celeste traveled much farther to her job, she was away from home much more than she used to be. Knowing that skin problems can be a bellwether for many things, I suggested that boredom and loneliness were the new factors that had upset Heidi's delicate balance.

Celeste realized that she was not spending as much time with Heidi as she used to and admitted that the dog was probably bored and lonely. We brainstormed, and Celeste decided to have somebody come in to play with the dog to offer her more companionship and activity. Once the new arrangement began, Heidi's allergies began to fade and she resumed her progress toward wellness.

Once you have chosen an individual animal, you need to take into account that dogs and cats require almost constant companionship and mental stimulation. We bring pets into our lives to help us meet some of our needs, but our lifestyles often deprive them of getting *their* needs met in turn. As I have learned from many years in my veterinary practice, **boredom and loneliness are probably the most damaging stress factors in a pet's life**. Animal behaviorists, such as Temple Grandin, agree. (See the Selected Bibliography in the Appendix.) Many pets are locked up alone for most of the days of their lives in our sensory-reduced, climate-controlled homes, cut off both from us and from the ebb and flow of natural and social life taking place outside the walls. When we come home, they may still have to wait while we attend to other obligations or pleasures. But being deprived of companionship, mental stimulation, and wholesome activity runs against the requirements of a dog or cat's nature and can lead to behavioral issues, such as barking, aggression, or withdrawal, as well as general health problems.

We are the dog's substitute for the pack and the cat's substitute for its community. When we take in a pet, we oblige ourselves to take on these responsibilities as best we can. There's no denying that doing so requires ongoing time and effort. If we can't manage it, our pets may show signs of negative stress by ripping at furniture, digging at carpets, barking at everything, chewing themselves raw, or becoming despondent. Others will learn to get through the deprivation by going unconscious—sleeping—most of the time. Not a great way to spend a life.

Being isolated is even more stressful for young animals. Puppies and kittens are born in groups that are meant to do everything together until they're nearly grown up. Animal parents would not leave a young litter—never mind a single infant—alone without protection, and would supply them with comfort, guidance, and an education in how to survive and relate socially. They would not expect them to grow up by themselves. Yet we often adopt very young puppies and kittens and expect them to tolerate being alone every day while we're away. Because

When You Adopt

When you adopt, you take responsibility for another living being's life. Take your decision seriously for both your sakes. Few things in life are as rewarding as seeing a beloved animal become trusting, happy, and well.

both dogs and cats adapt when they must, we may imagine that they're okay by themselves, but neither species copes well with these situations. Although cats can tolerate being alone somewhat better than dogs can, they need company and stimulation, too.

Animals need meaningful, *real* contact. If you already have a pet and must be out a lot, there's still much you can do. Properly run doggy daycares or day camps provide social satisfaction and an outlet for energy for many dogs. If you can't quite afford that kind of service, have a dog who doesn't mix well socially, or have cats, can you come home for lunch? If not, see whether an animal-loving friend, relative, or neighbor will regularly drop in to spend at least half an hour playing, stroking, or even just talking to your pet. A second pet may keep your first one company to an extent, but this won't meet all his needs. When you *are* home, include your pet in your activities and give him lots of attention. If you spend a lot of time watching TV, surfing the Net, or talking on the phone, he won't get what he needs. The animal in your care needs to be as important to you as he would be to his own kind.

Socialize Pets to Reduce Future Stress

Noodle, a golden doodle, was brought to a dog park for the first time when she was barely three months old. While she tried to get her bearings, a large black Labrador retriever bounded over the hill and ran at her. Even though the Lab didn't attack her, she was very frightened and hid behind Shannon, her person. The rambunctious behavior of a strange dog when she was too young to handle it left a strong impression. For the rest of her life, Noodle reacted to any similar dog that she met.

To become properly socialized, puppies and kittens must have gentle, friendly, regular contact with people, with their own kind, and with other species. Nothing can substitute for an early education in how to read and respond to the cues of the mixed community they'll be part of all their lives. While they're growing up they'll need a lot of social contact. Recently adopted adult animals also need to be brought into new situations in a caring and respectful way. But each animal's needs differ, so there's no golden rule for how to do this. Instead, we must do our best to try to figure out how and when to introduce each individual to new situations. For example, a dog or cat may be shy, outgoing, or somewhere in between. It's very important not to push an animal to do something he isn't ready to do. But even though his basic nature won't change, attentive and loving support will help him adapt and come into better balance with the multispecies, social world in which he must live.

Dogs in particular need guidance and limits to give them a sense of security and place. Canines teach their young everything they need to know about how to conduct themselves within the dynamics and expectations of the pack. As our dogs' substitute packs, we must teach them how to live among humans. If we don't, they may face serious consequences.

Understandably, some people are conflicted, even negative, about the idea of training their dogs because traditional methods were harsh and sometimes abusive, and they don't believe in treating vulnerable animals that way. But training need not be brutal or punitive; the best methods today take a much more subtle and respectful view of the dog's nature. And training must work *with* the individual and not against her. Do you have a busy Border collie who needs a playground of her own? An intense little terrier? A goofy Newfy? A laid-back greyhound who loves to watch TV? Be realistic about your pet's personality and

Resources for Socializing Dogs

Choose your trainer carefully; ask lots of questions and trust your gut feeling about whether this person and approach is right for you and your dog. The following experts offer different approaches for socializing (training) dogs. Their material can help you become aware of some of the perspectives available today.

Silvia Jay is an experienced dog behavior expert who teaches a noncoercive approach called Mindful Leadership. Contact her at: (902) 843-2182 or visit www.voice4dogs.com. Book: *Dump Dog*. Available from DogWise at (800) 776-2665 or dogwise.com.

Pat Miller is one of the leading trainers and developers of dog-friendly, positive methods. Contact her at: (301) 582-9420 or visit www.peaceablepaws.com. Books: *The Power of Positive Dog Training* and *Positive Perspectives: Love Your Dog, Train Your Dog*. Available from DogWise at (800) 776-2665 or dogwise.com.

For further information, see the Selected Resources in the Appendix.

seek out the most constructive and humane advice on how to train and socialize your beloved companion. Read some books. Do some research. But don't rely on books, television, or the Internet alone to guide you—you could seriously misjudge your dog's needs this way. Take some classes. Seek out an experienced trainer or canine behaviorist and get individual attention and advice for you, your dog, and the relationship you have with each other.

When You and Your Pet Share a Shelter

Fred and Ginger were a pair of long-haired cats who lived with my client Naomi and got along fine together. Then Naomi bought her dream condo. She believed the cats would prefer it physically to the old place, but this was not the case. They could hear a barking dog nearby, the street was busier, and the building was noisy. For those particular cats, these were all stress factors.

Ginger adapted well enough, but Fred did not and he started house-soiling and spraying to mark his territory. So Naomi came to me to ask what to do. It was a very challenging problem. Short of her selling the place, we tried to figure out which features in the cat's new situation she *could* adjust.

It happened that Naomi left Fred and Ginger alone a lot. In the old house, the cats had been fine with this, but in the new building Naomi's absence may have increased Fred's upset. Going on this theory, we gave the cats flower essences (see page 166) and Naomi arranged for somebody to come in during the day to play with them so they'd have something other than the new environment to focus on. Fred gradually stopped spraying and soiling, although he occasionally regressed. But Naomi was prepared to provide ongoing support to help him cope.

Your pet's needs for shelter may not always match yours. She may need to live and sleep in a cooler or warmer temperature than you. She may crave the natural, interesting sounds and scents of other animals and the world outside and be stressed out by loud music and other unnaturally amplified noise, as well as by artificial scents from room deodorizers and household maintenance products. A rugged breed that is traditionally used to the outdoors will typically suffer more stress from spending too much time inside than will a delicate breed raised for centuries to live indoors with its people. Think about how you can provide Esmeralda with ways to escape from too much, too little, or disturbing noise, scent, light, activity, temperature, and so on both inside and outside your home; consider how to increase her access to what she needs to make her feel alive, safe, and happy.

GO GREEN FOR PETS' SAKE

Did you know that dogs and cats are probably exposed to more pollution than we are? Their fur coats trap airborne and other pollutants,

Feeling Alive

Not everyone agrees that dogs and cats are capable of feeling self-consciously alive and happy. It's a subject that people debate from time to time, and one about which you must ultimately draw your own conclusion. However, I personally believe there's no question that animals feel happiness and joy, and that they take pleasure in being alive.

which they lick off. They live, breathe, eat from, and sleep on the ground where pollution collects. Pet food and toys come under minimal regulation compared to people's food and toys. Finally, public health warnings about product and chemical safety usually don't warn us of their danger to pets, even though their dangers to humans are often proven by tests on animals.

You can't protect your pet from all environmental stress, but you can take four steps that will make a big difference for her. Most important, support her living terrain with an unprocessed diet, balanced exercise, and a holistic approach toward her life needs and health care. The stronger her living terrain, the better she'll hold her own when facing environmental stress. Second, reduce her environmental stress as much as you can. Here are some ways to do this.

Industrial pollution. This is probably the worst environmental culprit. Become more aware of indoor and outdoor pollutants. *Chemical* pollution may be present in just about anything. Examples include drinking water, household cleaning products, pharmaceutical drugs, processed pet food, pet toys, household deodorizers, antiflea products, and synthetic building materials that may release toxic gases into your home for years. Some of the most common household pollutants include cigarette smoke, lead, pesticides, and formaldehyde, but there are many more.[1] When you can, use products that do not contain chemical pollutants.

Don't Wash Your Pet with People Shampoo

Did you know that shampoos and conditioners made for people—including baby shampoo—can irritate your pet's skin? Dogs and cats have higher skin pH levels than we do. Human skin is naturally acidic, whereas cats' is only slightly so, and dogs' is alkaline. Shampoos and conditioners adjusted for human skin are too acidic for dogs or cats, which may explain why some pets hate being bathed. Wrong pH products can also cause skin to flake and throw its normal bacterial flora off balance. This dysbiosis can lead to other problems.

Compare the pH levels below to see the difference between human, feline, and canine skin.[2]

Human skin	Feline skin	pH neutral	Canine skin
4.8 = acidic	6.4 = slightly acidic	7.0 = neutral	7.4 = alkaline

Use products made specifically for dogs or cats that state they've been adjusted to the correct pH level. Ideally, they should contain but a few simple ingredients and be as unprocessed as possible. If you can find them, aim for products that are free from industrial toxins, additives, and synthetic chemicals. For example, avoid detergent-based shampoos; although they create a nice foam they deplete fatty acids

Radiation pollution. This may come from microwaves, cell phones, two-way radios, computers, televisions, live electric cables in the wall, and so on. Place your pet's bedding, food and water bowls, and litter boxes at least a few feet away from electrical devices, even if they're in the next room and on the other side of a wall.

Polluted products. Although public health warnings often ignore animal health concerns, *you* don't have to. Keep products suspected of harming either people *or* animals out of your pet's domain. Examples include lead paints on imported toys and phthalate plasticizers in vinyls.

in the skin. Avoid insecticides such as pyrethrins found in flea and tick shampoos—use them only in rare cases of massive infestation, and never use pyrethrins near cats. As well, be alert to your pet's sensitivities, which you will discover through trial and error. For example, oatmeal may be wonderful for most individuals' skin, but some pets are allergic to it. If your choices are limited, select the best you can find and use it sparingly. Occasional use of a product containing industrial chemicals won't be the end of the world, especially if you support your pet's living terrain with a balanced, unprocessed diet.

DODGE THESE INGREDIENTS

Here's a starter list of shampoo and conditioner ingredients to avoid. They may be carcinogenic, immune disruptors, neurological disruptors, hormone disruptors, or reproductive toxicants. The list is not exhaustive.

PEG or polyethylene glycol; TEA or DEA; selenium sulfide; SLS, SLES, or sodium laureth sulfate; diethyl phthalate; iodopropynyl butylcarbamate; lecithin; resorcinol; FDC yellow 6; parabens; sodium lauryl sulfate; propylene glycol; tocopheryl acetate; and fragrance.[3] (See the Selected Bibliography in the Appendix for more information.)

(See Susan Weinstein's article, "Why Vinyl Stinks," listed in the Selected Bibliography section.)

House dust and dirt. More than mere fluff, house dust and dirt have been found to contain high concentrations of industrial pollution.[4] Because pets' fur coats trap dust and dirt and they live on the ground where it collects, they encounter it much more intimately than we do. Fortunately, thorough housekeeping—especially regular vacuuming and dusting—helps control household toxins. But conventional cleaning products may introduce more pollutants back into your home.

Instead, use organic or biodegradable household cleansers, yard and garden care products, and flea and other pest controls that support—rather than attack—the living terrain.

Choose Exercise That's Moderate, Balanced, and Safe

All things in moderation; your pet's exercise is no exception. Chasing after a flying disc might be a great occasional treat for your Scottie, but if he pursues this repetitive, high-impact activity day in and day out he could well end up with arthritis. In comparison, taking a dog through a well-rounded agility course may be a more balanced activity if it keeps the dog moving up, down, through, and around things and thus moves his limbs and muscles more evenly. Another form of exercise that, while exciting, can create negative stress is riding a bicycle while having the family dog run alongside. Pounding along on pavement is hard on anyone's bones; a dog doesn't have special jogging shoes designed to absorb shock. Also, no one can control the behavior of car drivers, even when the dog himself can be relied on to stay beside the bike. On the other hand, a brisk hike through hilly territory or along a dirt trail through the woods will provide a more natural terrain and keep a dog safe from cars. For every pet, exercise should create positive stress that leads to greater wellness, whereas too little or unsuitable activity can create negative stress and loss of wellness.

For dogs, playing or walking the territory together are two examples of exercise that tone the body while satisfying mental, social, and instinctual needs at the same time. Structured activities such as agility training or fly-ball practice are other examples. A dog may perform on an exercise machine to please you, but it won't fulfill him as would a real outing with you or perhaps with a regular dog walker he likes. A cat needs toys she can chase around the room, ideally with you tossing

Fresh Air

Recent studies have shown that air pollution may be worse inside our homes than outside them.[3] Fresh air helps clear out accumulated toxins and odors, changes the temperature of a room, and brings in the stimulating natural scents your pet needs. Unless you live in a very polluted town, try to let fresh air into your home whenever possible. If you cannot open your windows, you may be able to bring in fresh air with an air exchanger. Avoid the use of air fresheners and deodorizers, which may introduce more industrial chemicals into the indoor environment than are already present.

them or cheering her on, and better yet, a yard where she can feel the sun and the grass, breathe fresh air, and hear fascinating live noises while she moves about. Watching TV and batting at birds flying across the screen may provide a cat with occasional stimulation, but these distractions should not substitute for play with an actual companion every day. Although we humans may accept technological innovations as substitutes for real activities or relationships, animals need the real thing in order to thrive.

Too little or too much exercise. The amount of exercise your pet needs will differ from that of other pets. Some animals can exert themselves for long periods, while others tire easily due to normal constitutional differences or their level of wellness to begin with. Pushing an aging or arthritic individual too far or curbing an energetic pet who thrives on exercise will create negative stress with potentially serious consequences. Learn how much exercise your pet needs and can handle.

Age, disability, and your pet's exercise level. Young animals need more exercise while they develop physically, emotionally, and mentally. On the other hand, even the healthiest cat or dog will slow down as he gets older. Never push an old, arthritic, obese, or ill animal too hard. Too much exercise will stress him. Cats will refuse to

Be Present with Your Pet

If you're out walking with Fido or home rubbing the Monster Cat's chin, be *present* with your pet,—*especially* if he's been waiting hours for you to join him. Don't be mentally "elsewhere," such as talking on your cell phone. That may be fun for you, but it's not fair to Fido or the cat. Your pet needs socially meaningful, wholesome activity with you and other people or pets that he loves.

participate when they've had enough, but some dogs—such as those from the working breeds—may push *themselves* harder than is good for them. When you start to exercise a pet who isn't used to it, begin gently and gradually increase the time and intensity. Take special care with Weekend Warriors—the couch potato who rests quietly at home five days a week will be severely stressed if you take him out jogging on Saturday. Short walks or easy games are often enough for such animals. Use your best judgement, learn all you can about what's best for *your* pet, and know when to call it a day.

The needs of the breed. Different breeds have different energy levels and abilities and benefit from exercise through which they can express those abilities. For example, hunting and racing dogs are born to run; herding dogs to sprint, dodge, and turn; and retrievers to swim and fetch. Every breed requires moderate exercise; too much could create dangerous negative stress. Cats' abilities also vary, although most love games that tantalize their predatory instincts. But again, every pet remains an individual. For example, one golden retriever may be very laid-back and another a bundle of energy. Whether your pet loves to leap, pounce, run, climb, chase, fetch, or just trot proudly at your side, make sure that he gets enough of his favorite activities every day. And remember, as in the case of Samantha who spent most of her time at her computer until she adopted Newton, her Great Dane, doing what's best for your pet can also increase your own well-being.

A Diet That Supports the Living Terrain

When Susan adopted a four-year-old cat named Fulleh, the black domestic short-haired was in terrible shape. Fulleh weighed twenty-one pounds and was so obese she could hardly stand. When she tried to walk she would clump noisily across the room then roll over onto her side like a beached whale. Her hocks braced against each other to hold up her back end, and her belly dragged along the floor. Running, leaping, or any normal feline activity was clearly impossible for her. And that wasn't all. Her coat was dull, greasy, and prolific with dandruff; she shed too much; and tapeworm segments crept in and out of her anus. Fulleh was so fat she couldn't clean away the feces stuck to the hairs under her tail, and she was chronically constipated to boot. On top of everything else, she was constantly hungry and cried for food. By some miracle, she hadn't yet become diabetic, as obese cats commonly do.

Unfortunately, the woman who'd given Fulleh up had only been concerned about feeding her as cheaply as possible, and she had relied upon whatever loose kibble the local discount box store had emptied into the bargain bin. But inexpensive pet foods tend to be grain-based, low in meat, and high in carbohydrates, which I believe is exactly the opposite of what cats need to thrive. I've seen many cats such as Fulleh crave more and more of such food as they strive to fulfill their protein requirements, while simultaneously gaining weight from the carbohydrates they cannot properly digest.

Fulleh needed a jump-start to bring her back to wellness, so Susan brought her in for a standard veterinary dewormer. Then she put her on a diet of fresh, unprocessed meats with a little ground vegetable mixed in, along with pureed organic pumpkin to help reestablish normal bowel function. Thankfully, Fulleh was not a fussy eater and took to the new diet right away.

In the weeks and months that followed, Fulleh made a dramatic recovery. She lost weight and her belly started clearing the floor. Her fur became glossy and her dandruff faded away. Eventually, she became able to walk gracefully again, her hind legs straightened out, and she started jumping onto stools and chairs. Finally, she appeared not to be hungry all the time and stopped crying out for nourishment. An unprocessed diet gave Fulleh back her life.

Nothing as much as diet so greatly affects an animal's condition and ability to respond to stress. The living terrain depends on food for its nourishment. The way to support a dog or cat's living terrain is by providing a diet of fresh, species-appropriate, unprocessed food.

WHY *UNPROCESSED* FOOD?

If someone told you to eat processed food 365 days a year, no doubt you'd think he was crazy. Yet too often, this is exactly how we feed our pets. You probably know that processed foods aren't healthy for you and that you should eat at least *some* fresh food. A diet based on processed food cannot properly support a pet's living terrain any more than it can your own.

Processed food is any food that comes packaged in a bag or a can. It's processed to make it less biologically vital so it can be stored for a long time without deteriorating. Made for convenience, processed foods vary greatly in quality. The most problematic derive their protein from grains—an unnatural source for carnivores—and are high in carbohydrates, which carnivores don't handle very well, as authors such as Ian Billinghurst have pointed out. Many, including some of the more costly brands, are based on meat by-products that have little or no nutritional value. Processed food products frequently contain drug and pesticide residues, sugar, salt, and industrial dyes, flavorings, preservatives, and other pollutants and additives. (See the Selected Bibliography in the Appendix for more information.)

To be fair, some processed pet foods use higher quality, more expensive ingredients such as organic or otherwise choice meats and vegetables. These contain only natural preservatives, such as vitamins C and E, and no harmful, unnecessary additives. But because processing destroys so many nutrients, the manufacturer must reintroduce vitamins and minerals to the mix. Processing also diminishes the synergy between ingredients and the life energy that the food originally contained, and this cannot be recovered. So even the best processed foods are concoctions of modified and de-energized original foodstuffs and reintroduced isolated nutrients, a far cry from the whole, vital food the living terrain needs.

On the other hand, unprocessed foods are fresh, organic when possible, and in their original, unmodified states. Still biologically active, they are vibrant with energy and contain naturally balanced nutrients that work synergistically to nourish your pet's wellness. Although not as convenient as processed foods, they're much more suitable to support the living terrain. You may serve them raw, or cook them gently if you or your pet prefer. Because they consist of natural ingredients in their original format, they typically contain fewer pollutants and additives than processed foods do. You may compromise a *little* and give your pet both processed and unprocessed food, but you must emphasize the unprocessed kind. (There are many books that make excellent cases for the superiority of feeding pets an unprocessed diet; see the Selected Bibliography in the Appendix.)

One justification for processing food is that it eliminates unfriendly bacteria and renders the food less habitable for new bacterial growth. However, food processing mixes components from many sources, and these components are handled by many people in different manufacturing plants. Before they end up in our hands they have numerous opportunities to become tainted with industrial toxins. This is the

If You Can Cook for Yourself . . .

Most of us believe we can prepare a proper diet for our children and ourselves. How, then, have we come to believe that we're not capable of doing the same for our cats and dogs? One possible reason is that pet food companies, given their need to sell products, may promote the impression that they alone can prepare a properly balanced diet for pets. This implies that pet owners aren't capable of feeding pets properly on their own. If we can feed our kids and ourselves just fine every day, *surely* we can do the same for our dogs and cats.

heartbreaking lesson of the pet food tragedies of 2007 that made many people aware for the first time of the complexities of food processing. We learned that we can't know the journey that most processed foods have taken, and we can't guarantee that every contributor along the line has our pets' best interests in mind.

Unprocessed foods run less risk of industrial contamination; if you source them directly by growing your own vegetables or buying meats directly from farmers, you can limit that risk even more. But because they're biologically active, they're more susceptible to organic contamination from unfriendly bacteria and the like. They may decay very quickly, so every handler, including you, must keep them fresh and away from contaminants. Choose the best natural foodstuffs you can afford. Aim to buy meats and vegetables that have been least exposed to chemicals, pesticides, or drugs (including those given to farm animals such as antibiotics and growth hormones). Meats that come from pasture-raised animals are excellent.

Making our pets' food ourselves may be more expensive and less convenient than taking prepared food from a shelf. However, people are becoming more aware of the value of unprocessed food and the long-term cost savings of having a healthier pet who has less need for expensive veterinary attention. As well, the pet food scare of 2007 made

The Melamine Tragedies of 2007 and 2008

In 2007, when melamine and other toxic industrial chemicals turned up in hundreds of pet foods, reliable sources at the time reported that thousands of beloved dogs and cats were killed and countless others damaged.[6] As if this warning bell weren't enough that manufacturers could contaminate the food supply, melamine turned up again in 2008—this time in infant formula—and sickened possibly more than 300,000 human babies in China.[7] In this case, the toxin found its way into formula through not one but dozens of different upstream manufacturers.[8]

The presence of inappropriate stressors in the food supply has become an everyday concern for pets and people alike. You can significantly reduce the risk of contamination from manufacturing practices by providing your pet with unprocessed foods that you prepare from scratch. If you want to chew on a full account of how the globalization of the food supply creates dangers for both pets and people, read *Pet Food Politics* by Marion Nestle. (See the Selected Bibliography in the Appendix.)

people more wary of processed foods. As a consequence, a whole new cottage industry has emerged to make unprocessed food more conveniently available and less expensive.

Unprocessed pet food in convenient packaging is now available for purchase from natural pet supply shops. Made primarily of high-quality meat, it comes frozen and is often already balanced with vegetables and sometimes with nutritional supplements. It is also often customized to meet the needs of both dogs and cats of different ages and sometimes of different breeds. The amount to feed will depend upon your pet's weight, age, and activity level. Complete the diet with further supplements if advised by a holistic veterinarian. However, it's most economical to prepare unprocessed pet food yourself—plus, you can better control what's in it.

As you strive to care for your pet in the best possible way, remember that you can't change everything by yourself. For example, you may wish to provide pasture-fed meat but have no access to it. Or you may not be able to afford organic food for yourself and so cannot afford it for your pet, either. Just do the best you can; every little bit helps.

For my clinic's guidelines for an unprocessed diet for dogs and cats, see The Stress-Busters Diet for Dogs and Cats in the Appendix.

Immunization and Stress

Many years ago, I followed mainstream vaccination protocol. This involved using a number of different vaccines and injecting them all on the same day. One day, some clients brought in a healthy, temperamentally balanced young puppy. When I gave him his injection he yelped, ran across the office floor, and whimpered in the corner for a long time. Eventually, his owners decided to take him home and allow him to recover there. But from the day of that injection onward, that puppy became afraid of everything. In fact, he did not recover.

In another case, right after I gave a dog a routine vaccination he went into anaphylactic shock. While his people looked on in horror, we tried desperately to save him, but he died within minutes right on the table in front of us. These tragic incidents caused me to question the accepted approach to immunization.

I set about studying the issue, and as a result we stripped down our immunization schedule to a bare minimum. We also stopped assuming that our patients needed boosters every year, and instead began monitoring their immunity levels with antibody tests. Since we implemented this stringent new protocol, our patients have had no further dramatic negative reactions.

Immunization is a mixed bag. On the positive side, it has been extremely effective in protecting pets from infectious diseases. For example, when I first started practice in 1962 and vaccines either didn't exist or weren't widely available, I saw many, many cases of canine distemper, and I don't want to go back to those days. So I don't entirely rule it out. But on the worrisome side, vaccination is a significant stressor that attacks the living terrain and gives pets' immune systems a beating. As a result, it has created serious new health problems that can range from immediate and potentially fatal reactions such as anaphylactic shock to long-lasting behavioral changes.[9] These problems should make us very cautious when it comes to vaccinating pets.

Here are some of my concerns with immunization.

Overimmunization. Puppies and kittens come into the world with specific innate immunities that their mothers gave them, and they are meant to increase these innate immunities as they grow. In contrast, vaccination creates artificially acquired immunity. Recent research has found that if the acquired immunity that we impose upon young animals is excessive, it stops them from developing their innate immunities as they are meant to do.[10] Although what is excessive to each individual will vary, the traditional immunization protocol, which is arbitrary and anything but minimal, sets up the context in which overimmunization can happen.

Forcing disease into the living terrain. Vaccines intentionally introduce disease into the living terrain. They work by creating latent subterranean disease—a low level of disease that remains hidden beneath the surface—to provoke the body to develop antibodies against it. But the living terrain isn't meant to have harmful foreign material forced into it in such a way. This artificial disease process can backfire on some individuals, and may show up as a subtle, hard to define malaise. (See Chapter 5.) When evaluating the usefulness of vaccines, we must consider not only the good they may do, but also the harm they may do.

Processed products with harmful additives. Vaccines contain not only the virus they inoculate against but also other ingredients. For example, they are commonly manufactured with additives intended to artificially stimulate a stronger immune response. These additives often consist of toxins known to be harmful to pets, such as mercury or other heavy metals.[11] In addition, the manufacturing process can cause ingredients to behave differently; this, in turn, can produce by-products that remain in the vaccine.[12] Vaccines may contain other contaminants as well.

A BETTER APPROACH

As I stated earlier, at my clinic we have had excellent results giving a bare minimum of vaccinations. Instead of starting pets off with a series of shots, we inoculate each animal only twice. And rather than using seven, eight, or more vaccines, we immunize against two diseases for dogs and two for cats. (See page 114.) Instead of following up with annual boosters, we assess our patients' immunity by taking titers, which are blood tests that measure antibody levels. As of this writing, we do more titers than any other veterinary clinic in Canada.

Since we initiated this protocol in the late 1990s, we've found that more than 98 percent of our patients maintain such high antibody levels that they never need a vaccination again. We've had such overwhelming success that we switched from doing titers annually to doing them every three years, with the same results. We see about 2,500 dogs every year, and titer about 500 of them. Of these, fewer than ten will need a booster. We have not seen a case of distemper for years except in a dog who had not been vaccinated against it (see Caleb's story beginning on page 157), and the most recent parvo cases I've seen were in dogs who had been vaccinated according to traditional protocol before they came to my clinic. We have had similar results with cats.

Our very successful approach has been largely influenced by the work of immunology experts Ron Schultz[13] and Jean Dodds[14], who have produced some of the best research showing the dangers of vaccines and that minimal immunization does protect against infectious

About the Cost of Titers

The cost of titering is more expensive than the cost of vaccinating, and some clients worry that it will be prohibitive. But we've found this not to be the case. Titering once every three years for the two diseases I recommend brings the price of titering close to the cost of vaccinating yearly against a large number of viruses. You can further reduce the amount you will pay for titering by asking to have it done when your pet is having blood taken for other kinds of tests. This way, you'll only need to pay for one office visit and one fee for extracting blood.

diseases. However, we have had marvelous results using even fewer vaccines and fewer injections than they recommend.[15] (See the Selected Resources in the Appendix for more on Schultz and Dodds's work.)

HOW TO IMMUNIZE FOR MAXIMUM BENEFIT AND MINIMAL STRESS

The following immunization schedules are given with the understanding that those who follow them also support their pets' living terrain in the ways I describe in this book. A healthy living terrain is the best protection against infectious diseases.

Schedule for puppies and kittens. Vaccinate the young of both species only twice. Ideally, they should receive the first shot at nine weeks of age (or at least two weeks after nursing ends—whichever comes *later*) and the second one at sixteen weeks (or seven weeks after the first one; whichever comes *later*). However, it's common to adopt a six- or seven-week-old puppy or kitten who has already been vaccinated. To ensure that these youngsters still receive a vaccination close to the crucial nine-week-old point, they should receive another shot three weeks after their original one (and *no sooner*). For example, if a pet was seven weeks old when he had his first vaccination, he should

Rabies Vaccinations Should Follow Suit

Most regions have legislation requiring that dogs, and sometimes cats, be vaccinated against rabies either annually or once every three years. But the duration of immunity of rabies vaccinations is currently under study, and I believe that up-to-date research will likely show they are fully effective when given every five years or even less frequently[16]. Although I do not advise you to violate the law, I look forward to the day when, on behalf of animal wellness, the law will reflect the scientific research on this subject. How long that might take is anyone's guess.

have another at ten weeks, and then the last one (seven weeks later) at seventeen weeks of age. Although these animals will receive a total of three vaccinations rather than the two that I consider ideal, I believe this revised schedule will significantly enhance their immunity. **If a puppy or kitten reacts negatively to any vaccine, never give it to him again.**

Once your kitten or puppy has completed this minimal immunization protocol, you can do a blood test to measure his immunity any time after two weeks following the final inoculation. I usually do the first titer one year after a youngster has received his final vaccine at sixteen weeks.

Which vaccines. My clinic vaccinates dogs only against canine distemper virus and canine parvovirus. We vaccinate cats only against feline panleukopenia and feline viral rhinotracheitis (FVR). Unfortunately, each of these pairs of vaccines is usually combined together during manufacture. As a general rule, I believe it's better for the immune system to receive only one vaccine at a time, but when they are not available as single vaccines, and allowing that my clinic's immunization protocol is so minimal, I do give these as combinations. Our patients have not shown any significant problems receiving these vaccines in combination since we reduced the frequency and type of vaccinations that we give overall.

If you have a pet who has been overvaccinated. If your dog or cat has been vaccinated according to the traditional protocol I described earlier, then in my opinion he has been overvaccinated. Before he receives another booster, have a titer done to check his immunity for the two viruses that pertain to his species which I specified earlier. A titer will give you a count for the presence of antibodies in your pet's system, and your vet will be able to tell you whether the count is sufficient to provide immunity against these diseases. If it is, your pet will not need a vaccination at this time. From then on, titer every three years. Your pet may never need another vaccination again. However, until the laws change to reflect a similar protocol concerning rabies, you will still be required to immunize against rabies.

At the discretion of the veterinarian, homeopathic Thuja or Silicea could be helpful to support the living terrain immediately following vaccination.

Even when you have done everything you can to support your pet's living terrain, at times your cat or dog may still become unwell and therefore vulnerable to disease. This is why holistic thinking regards *unwellness* as a matter of great importance to both short-term and long-term health outcomes. Fortunately, there's lots you can do to help your pet, starting with learning how to identify the early signs of unwellness.

ENDNOTES

1. "Dangerous Chemicals in the Home: A Most-Wanted List of Five Common Household Contaminants," Natural Resources Defense Council (NRDC), www.nrdc.org/health/home/fchems.asp (accessed January 4, 2009).

2. Jennifer L. Matousek and Karen L. Campbell, "A Comparative View of Cutaneous pH," *Veterinary Dermatology* 13, no. 6 (December 2002): 293–300.

3. Drawn from the Environmental Working Group (www.ewg.org) and the Natural Skincare Authority (www.natural-skincare-authority.com/hair-shampoo-toxins.html), both accessed December 22, 2008; and an interview with Kim Green, groomer and pet care consultant.

4. Sonja Renee, "PBDEs—Fire Retardants in Dust: Toxic Fire Retardants in American Homes," Environmental Working Group Research, May 2004, www.ewg.org.

5. U.S. Environmental Protection Agency, "The Inside Story: A Guide to Indoor Air Quality," U.S. EPA/Office of Air and Radiation, Office of Radiation and Indoor Air (6609J), Cosponsored with the Consumer Product Safety Commission, EPA 402-K-93-007.

6. "Melamine Contamination Killed Thousands of Pets, Says a New Report," *Bio-Medicine.org*, latest biology and medical news/technology, April 10, 2007, www.bio-medicine.org/medicine-news/Melamine-Contamination-Killed-Thousands-of-Pets—Says-a-New-Report-19774-1/; "Brothers Charged over Tainted Baby Milk," Canadian Broadcasting Company, September 15, 2008, www.cbc.ca/health/story/2008/09/15/tainted-milk.html.

7. "China's Tainted-milk Toll Rises to 300,000 Sick Children," Canadian Broadcasting Company, December 2, 2008, www.cbc.ca/health/story/2008/12/02/china-babies.html.

8. "Food Recalls Grow in Chinese Tainted Milk Crisis," Canadian Broadcasting Company, September 25, 2008, www.cbc.ca/world/story/2008/09/25/chinese-recalls.html.

9. W. Jean Dodds, "Vaccination Protocols for Dogs Predisposed to Vaccine Reactions," *Journal of the American Animal Hospital Association* 38 (2001): 1–4.

10. W. Jean Dodds, "Complementary and Alternative Veterinary Medicine: The Immune System," *Clinical Techniques in Small Animal Practice* 17, no. 1 (February 2002): 58–63.

11. Mattie J. Hendrick et al, "Postvaccinal Sarcomas in the Cat: Epidemiology and Electron Probe Microanalytical Identification of Aluminum," *Cancer Research* 52 (1992): 5391-94; Keitaro Ohmori et al, "IgE Reactivity to Vaccine Components in Dogs That Developed Immediate-type Allergic Reactions After Vaccination," *Veterinary Immunology and Immunopathology* 104 (2005): 249–56.

12. E. Katheryn Myer, "Vaccine-associated Adverse Effects," *Veterinary Clinics of North America: Small Animal Practice* 31 (2001): 493–514.

13. Ronald D. Schultz, "Current and Future Canine and Feline Vaccination Programs," *Veterinary Medicine* 93, no. 3 (March 1998): 233–54.
14. W. Jean Dodds, "More Bumps on the Vaccine Road," *Advances in Veterinary Medicine* 41 (1999): 715–32.
15. We vaccinate our patients more minimally than Schultz recommends. In Schultz's protocol, puppies and kittens would receive a third vaccination at eleven or twelve weeks of age (timed to take place between the two that my clinic administers). He also advises that dogs receive CAV-2 vaccine. However, my clinic has had great success without these additional measures.
16. "Why Challenge Current Rabies Vaccine Policy?," Rabies Challenge Fund, www.rabieschallengefund.org/page4.html (accessed January 8, 2009).

PART THREE

Assessing Unwellness

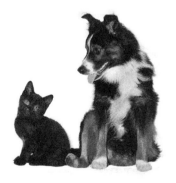

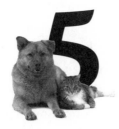

Learn the Early Signs, Then Trust Your Instincts

Checkers, a black and white domestic short-haired cat, belonged to a working couple who had no children. When Checkers was six years old, Anne and Sabah moved from their old house to a new condominium in a building still under construction. Soon after the move, they began to notice that Checkers's behavior had changed. Although he'd always been outgoing and friendly, now he often hid, and when he did come out to spend time with them he seemed anxious and demanded lots of attention. And instead of using his litter box he began to relieve himself on the floor beside it, something he had never done before.

One day, blood appeared in his urine. Checkers's vet diagnosed him with a bladder infection and put him on antibiotics. His infection seemed to clear up, but he still wouldn't use his litter box or otherwise behave like his old self. A few weeks later, the illness returned. After another round of antibiotics it disappeared again, but following this Checkers lost enthusiasm for his food. When the infection returned a third time, Anne and Sabah felt that the diagnosis they had received did not explain the entire picture. Wanting to try a different approach, they brought the cat to me for another opinion.

First, I confirmed that Checkers's bacterial infection had returned; that part was easy. But although it needed attention, from a holistic point of view it was not the cat's main issue. More important was that something had stressed out his living terrain and made him unwell and therefore vulnerable to bacterial illness in the first place. To solve the problem, we first had to figure out what had caused the cat's original loss of wellness.

To investigate Checkers's present life circumstances, I started with the most obvious stressful event. Moving from a familiar place to an unfamiliar one is psychologically hard on pets and often brings other stressors with it. So I asked the clients, "What's different about where you used to live compared to where you live now?"

Anne said, "Our old place was a house, but now we live in an apartment. It's brand new—the units down the hall from us are still under construction."

Here was our first clue. Loud noises can be very stressful to pets, especially if the animal is in a strange place. "It must be noisy," I said.

"It is," Anne said, "but we don't hear it that often. We're gone during the day."

Here was another possible clue. Perhaps the cat was being left alone more often than he used to be. To find out, I asked, "Did you have the same schedule when you lived at your old house?"

Sabah answered, "Not really. We live farther away from work so we leave earlier and come back later each day. And Anne used to go home for lunch, but that's not possible anymore."

So along with the stress of the move and the jarring sounds of construction, Checkers probably also suffered from boredom and loneliness because now he was left alone most of the day. But we still needed to figure out why he had changed his litter habits.

Sabah explained that Checkers had begun to go outside his litter box after they bought him a new one and began to fill it with a different kind of litter. Checkers had lost his familiar box and may not like the new one.

Finally, I inquired about his appetite and learned that he'd always been a good eater until now.

Anne and Sabah had now described enough to explain Checkers's disrupted energy and loss of wellness. First, he had lost his familiar surroundings and found himself in a strange place. Then his litter box had been replaced with a new one that he didn't like and litter that he didn't want to stand in. Losing the old litter box also meant he'd lost an important source of continuity that might have helped him adjust to his new home. As well, when Anne and Sabah started leaving earlier, returning later, and not coming home for lunch, Checkers lost social contact and mental stimulation during the day. Add to this the loud noises and physical vibrations caused by major construction in the same building and from which he could not escape, and I thought we had a bead on the stress that had caused his unwellness.

In turn, Checkers's unwellness would explain why he had become vulnerable to a bladder infection—the stress that caused the unwellness would have impaired his immune system somewhat. Therefore, unfriendly bacteria had been able to overwhelm his living terrain and infected his bladder.

Following this development, the antibiotics he'd been prescribed had further complicated his condition. It wasn't *wrong* to use antibiotics; it's just that they didn't deal with the whole picture. Although they wiped out his bladder infection, they didn't address the negative stress that was its underlying cause, so his living terrain remained vulnerable to the infection's return. In relation to the antibiotics, iatrogenic stress—stress caused by medical intervention—and dysbiotic stress also played roles. Because antibiotics disrupt normal digestive bacteria, they can cause dysbiotic stress—imbalance in the intestinal flora— which probably explained the cat's loss of interest in food.

His case would have been quite different if a holistic approach had been followed instead. An orientation that favors methods that support the living terrain would not use antibiotics as a first line of defense but only as a last resort. So Checkers probably would not have been given antibiotics, and therefore would probably not have developed the dysbiotic stress that led to his loss of appetite.

To improve Checkers's level of wellness we had to improve his environment, so we talked about what Anne and Sabah might be able to do for him. Although they couldn't fix everything, they could reduce a lot of the negative stress in his life. First, they would put back his old litter box and the type of litter he preferred. Once he was completely secure in his new home, they could experiment with changing the litter again, but not until then.

Next, they would ask Sabah's aunt, a cat lover who Checkers liked and who lived in the area, if she could drop by every couple of days to spend a half hour with Checkers. If this didn't work out, they would hire a pet sitter or responsible young person to come by for regular visits when they were at work. When they were at home they would focus on spending time with Checkers and would try not to go out after work too often over the next few weeks while they helped him adjust to his new environment.

They couldn't do much about the construction noise, so they decided to leave on a classical music radio station when they were out. Checkers liked classical music, and at least its familiar sounds and rhythms might help ease him through the raucous sounds of the equipment next door. They also planned to place another bed for him in a quiet corner of the room farthest from the construction.

To support Checkers's living terrain I recommended a natural flower remedy to calm him, plus probiotics containing friendly, appropriate bacteria to help his digestive system recover from the effects of the antibiotics. To deal with his bladder infection, I started him on a couple of homeopathic remedies. I was sure he would be fine; he just needed extra support while he adapted.

A week later, Sabah called to say that Checkers had improved. He had started using his old litter box as soon as they gave it back to him, and after only a few days on the probiotics his appetite had returned to normal. His bladder infection was now clearing up on its own. Most important, he seemed to be much happier. Taken all together, his signs and symptoms had begun to recede and his living terrain appeared to be returning to homeostasis—the state of wellness.

Checkers's story shows that negative stress causes the unwellness that both leads to and *underlies* illness. This explains why antibiotics, homeopathics, and any other remedies—whether mainstream or otherwise—are not the final answer to a health problem. They may help a dog or cat in the short run, if used in an appropriate way at the optimal time. But simply *treating* illness is not enough. To really help a pet we must deal with her unwellness, which means finding and addressing the hidden stress that's causing it.

Checkers's story also shows how finding the stressor that's causing the problem can be like doing detective work to figure out who broke into the house. As we proceed we know we are looking for culprits, but our question is where to find them. We have to work from one clue to another. And the job doesn't end when we find a culprit—we also have to address how it gained a foothold in the first place. If we don't, another culprit may come along at a later time and rob the house again. Only in this way can we prevent illness from recurring.

Unfortunately, no matter how hard we try, we can't keep our pets well one hundred percent of the time. In our complicated world dogs and cats face all kinds of negative stressors, and sometimes they won't feel well. But we don't need to wait until an animal is sick to keep her from losing optimal wellness. By learning the signs of *unwellness* and dealing with the stress that's causing it, we can head off trouble *before* it turns into full-blown illness. And if she does become ill, we can not only help her overcome it but also reduce the chance that it will return.

Wellness, Unwellness, and Illness

If you're not sure of the difference between unwellness and illness or you've always believed that someone is either sick or healthy, then you're not alone. After all, good health was traditionally defined by mainstream medicine as the absence of disease. So the media, advertising, and many physicians still often take disease as their starting point. Mainstream physicians who follow this traditional concept of health tend to see patients as either ill or not ill, with little gray area in between, and they do not take action until a patient shows clear signs of illness. Under the influence of this kind of thinking, no wonder it can be hard to recognize that there's a lot more to wellness than being sick or not sick. Thank goodness mainstream medicine is also catching on to the importance of wellness rather than focusing only on illness.

Holistic thinking defines good health not as the absence of disease, but as the presence of full and radiant wellness. Because it takes wellness, instead of disease, as its starting point, it's able to see what the mainstream perspective tends to miss: *the road to illness is paved by loss of wellness.* Holistic veterinarians don't wait for signs of illness to appear, but begin to act as soon as a patient starts to lose wellness. From this perspective, waiting until illness sets in before taking action is like closing the barn door after the horse has left—the living terrain is already compromised and less able to recover from negative stress.

The holistic way understands that pets don't get sick all of a sudden; instead, they gradually lose wellness until they're no longer able to fend off a negative stressor and so become vulnerable to disease. It recognizes that health and illness are not cut-and-dried, on-or-off conditions. Instead, it relates to health as a spectrum that has wellness at one pole, illness at the opposite pole, and the loss of wellness—*unwellness*—stretching between the two. We can use the following definitions for these three realms of health.

Wellness = The presence of full-flowing energy and a strong and resilient living terrain that can bounce back and increase its wellness after being challenged by negative stress.

Unwellness = The subtle loss of wellness that begins long before a pet shows clear signs of illness and that is characterized by blocked energy, subtle symptoms, and a weakened response to stress.

Illness = A condition of obvious distress, characterized by clear signs and concrete evidence, in which negative stress has overwhelmed the living terrain.

The Importance of Unwellness

Because problem stress shows up as unwellness *before* it turns into illness, by understanding unwellness and learning how to recognize it you will gain several powerful advantages in taking care of your pet. You'll be able to tell when negative stress affects her before she gets sick. You'll have a chance to figure out which stressor has caused the problem and do something about it. When illness does develop, you'll be able to help prevent it from coming back. And the best part is, recognizing unwellness is not hard to do. It simply requires using your six senses; trust what you see and feel; pay attention to changes in your pet's appearance, behavior, habits, and even the way she smells; and consider whether these could be the early signs and symptoms of unwellness. For example, Checkers's people noticed that he was hiding a lot, had become needy of attention, and was relieving himself outside his box. If they had also recognized that these were signs of stress that could lead to unwellness, they would have known to look for solutions to his problems before he became ill.

THE EARLY SIGNS AND SYMPTOMS OF UNWELLNESS

The first thing to remember about unwellness is that it makes itself known through subtle, nonspecific signs, as opposed to illness, which usually makes itself known through clear, obvious signs. So, the clues to unwellness depend on how much you fine-tune your ability to notice them. But first, you need to have a detailed idea of what is normal for your cat or dog, so you'll be able to identify and describe any deviations from it. Plus, the better you can describe your pet's unwellness to yourself, the better you can communicate it to your veterinarian if you decide to seek out his help.

To observe your pet's unwellness, you'll need to ask yourself the kinds of questions I ask my clients when they bring their pets into my clinic.

Your Pet's General Habits

The first set of questions is very general. They cover your pet's sleeping habits, energy, appetite, and mood and behavior. Treat these and the questions about bodily functions that follow them as examples to get you thinking, and don't hesitate to note any changes that aren't listed here. Observe what's normal for her behavior, then note what has *changed.* You're not evaluating whether she's an avid eater or a fussy one, or whether she's outgoing or shy. You're looking for signs of whether she's begun to behave differently from what's normal for *her.*

Sleeping habits. Have your pet's sleeping habits changed recently? Does she sleep more than she used to? Or has she become restless at night?

Energy. Is your pet less energetic than usual? Does she seem tired or less responsive to you? Has she lost enthusiasm for activities she would normally enjoy, such as going for walks or playing with her favorite toys? Alternatively, has she become hyperactive compared to her normal self?

Appetite. How is your pet's appetite? Does she seem less interested in food? Does she turn away from her favorite treats? Or does she keep asking for more and seem anxious that she isn't getting enough?

Mood and behavior (when she's alone as well as in social interactions). Has your pet begun to relieve herself in the house, if she normally did not do that? Has she started to lick obsessively, scratch, or chew at her own body? Has she become more aggressive toward other people or pets, or more withdrawn? Does she seek your attention more? Has she begun defying your wishes, more than she used to? Has she begun trying to escape a room, the house, or the yard when she did not do this before?

Your Pet's Bodily Functions

The more detail you can give your vet about your pet's bodily functions, the better.

Coughing. Has your pet started coughing? Is it a dry cough, or does it produce mucus? What does her cough sound like? When, where, and how often does she cough?

Sneezing. Has she been sneezing? If so, once in a while, or often? Does she sneeze many times at once? Is her nose dripping? Is her mucus clear or milky? Do her eyes run?

Vomiting. Has your pet been vomiting lately? Does it happen after eating a meal, after eating certain foods, or does it seem to be unrelated to meals and snack times? Does it contain clear mucus, or is it more substantial?

Diarrhea or constipation. Your pet's stools are an instructive indicator of his overall condition. Have they been abnormal for longer than a day or two? Are they soft and loose, or harder and drier than usual? Is he going more often or less so? Does their color seem off, and do they smell strange or unusually strong? Do they contain undigested food, blood, mucus, or anything else that shouldn't be there?[1]

Weight change. Has your pet gained or lost weight recently, for reasons that aren't obvious?

Skin. Your pet's skin and coat are like neon signs that reflect the condition of her living terrain. Is she scratching a lot? Has her skin become dry? Has it become red and warm or hot to the touch? Does she have areas that are leathery, oozing, or blistered? Does she have cysts growing between her toes? Does she lick at her legs a lot, and have open sores where she licks? Has her coat become dull or has her hair begun to fall out?

Urinary. Has your pet begun urinating more often? Less often? Does he seem to have difficulty when he goes? Does the color seem off? Is he drinking more than usual?

Musculoskeletal. Is your pet limping? Has she begun hesitating to go up or down stairs? Do ordinary movements such as getting up or lying down seem difficult for her? If you run your hand lightly over her back and legs, do you notice unusual warmth coming from any of her joints or anywhere along her spine? Does she have trouble putting a foot down, or is the rhythm of her gait irregular in other ways?

If you suspect that your pet may be unwell, think about what kind of stress could be the underlying cause. Take into account every circumstance of her life at the moment. Rely on your six senses. Consider the eight realms of stress. Keep in mind the three conditions for your pet's wellness and assess whether she has a need that's not being met. In most cases you'll soon figure out what's bothering her, and you'll be glad you did.

WHEN TO TAKE YOUR UNWELL PET TO THE VET

When your pet is unwell, you will sometimes figure out for yourself what's causing his stress and correct it so he can recover. But other times you won't be able to determine on your own what is wrong or know what to do about it. When should you take your pet to the vet?

It's easier to know the answer to this question when an animal is *ill*. Guidelines for when to take an ill pet to the vet typically include the signs to look for and how quickly you should seek help. But for *unwell* pets, the guidelines aren't straightforward. There's no magic indicator such as, "If your pet vomits three times, call your vet." It's hard to put a timeline on how long to tolerate signs of unwellness before getting professional advice. So how do you decide?

Trust your instincts. You have to make the judgement call; it's up to you. You *know* when it's time to get advice. It may be when you have run out of ideas, or when nothing you do has made a difference. Or you might just *feel* it. At these times, take control of the situation. And take heart. Remember, you know your pet better than anyone.

Look for *persistent* early signs and symptoms of unwellness. For example, your pet may have low energy that doesn't seem to pick up again when you think it should. Or her appetite may change and not go back to normal. If you observe something abnormal or unusual that persists beyond a time you think is reasonable, it's time to consult a professional. And be sure to describe all your observations to your vet.

***Don't wait* until your pet becomes ill.** The best thing you can do for an unwell pet is get help for her *before* she becomes ill. Doing so may save her from a peck of trouble down the road. Don't worry about whether you're going to your vet too often or with symptoms that are too subtle to be worth mentioning. Remember that your vet is a coach who is available for you to consult with. He should not ignore small or nonspecific symptoms and your concern should prompt him to take the matter seriously. For example, if Checkers's people had consulted with me earlier about the subtle changes that he exhibited, we might have eased his stress enough to prevent him from developing a bladder infection in the first place. Protect your pet. Learn the signs and symptoms of unwellness, and get help before the situation gets worse.

When You See Signs of *Illness*

When an animal has been injured or shows signs of outright illness, she needs qualified help as soon as possible. A few possible signs of illness include blood in the stool or urine, trouble passing stool or urine, fever, an unfamiliar lump, and discharge from the eyes or nose. Keep yourself very well informed about signs of illness and emergencies.

What if your vet thinks there's nothing wrong, and you don't agree? Get a second opinion. You will need to decide whose approach to follow—especially if one vet thinks more holistically and the other has a mainstream orientation. Get all the information you can from both veterinarians, but don't expect either one to give you the answer. *You* decide which approach sounds right for your dog or cat and follow through with it. (See Selected Resources in the Appendix.)

Once you and your unwell pet arrive at the clinic, you'll face another challenge. Standard tests can detect illness, but not unwellness. Fortunately, as you'll see in the next chapter, a new field of scientific tests offers new options.

ENDNOTES

1. For a detailed discussion of how to "read" your dog's feces for signs of health issues, see Susan Weinstein, "Dog Gone Dung: Familiarity with Your Dog's Poop Will Help You Detect Illness Quickly," *The Whole Dog Journal* 9, no. 10 (October 2006): 14–19.

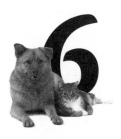

Working with Your Vet

When Jennifer brought Jesse, her four-year-old Shetland sheepdog, into my examination room, the dog showed no sign of illness. But Jennifer was sure he wasn't well. So I asked her a number of questions to determine whether she had observed any subtle signs of unwellness.

I began by asking whether he had his usual degree of enthusiasm for routine activities.

"He doesn't go upstairs or outside as often. He's been resting more than usual these days," Jennifer responded with concern. "He's still happy to go for his walk to the park, but when he's there he doesn't want to play with the other dogs for as long as he usually does."

"And how's he been sleeping?"

"Not soundly," she said. "He seems a bit restless."

"What about his appetite? Have you noticed any changes there?"

"He normally eats all his food, but these days he's been leaving some behind in the bowl. That's not like him."

Finally, I asked how Jesse seemed to be doing emotionally.

"I think he's kind of down," she said. "He lies around with his head on his paws. He's not smiling. This is partly how I noticed something was wrong in the first place. He's usually full of mischief."

Jennifer had observed some subtle signs of unwellness, which prompted me to investigate further. We ran some standard tests, including blood work and urinalysis, but the results showed no abnormalities. At this point, if we were thinking in a mainstream way, we might say, "This dog is fine." But Jennifer didn't think so. Following my conviction that the client knows her pet best, I suggested that bioenergetic assessment would help us find out more about Jesse's unwellness and the underlying stressor that was causing it. Jennifer agreed and we made an appointment for electrodermal screening the following week. I asked her to bring in samples of everything Jesse ate and any supplements that she normally gave him.

When the pair came back, Jennifer told me that in the week since his last appointment, Jesse had developed on-and-off diarrhea and his ears had become smelly. Obviously, Jennifer's sense that her dog was unwell had proved correct.

We went into the quiet staff lounge where we do bioenergetic assessments. Jesse got up on the sofa and Jennifer sat down beside him. We gave Jennifer a metal probe and directed her to gently place it against the pads of Jesse's paw and hold it there with her hand, so she could act as a vector for Jesse's energy. In her other hand, we placed a plastic bag containing some of Jesse's regular dog food. As Jesse's energy field reacted to the sample, the probe relayed the change to the computer, which registered numbers on the screen. Then we replaced the bag of dog food with a sample of Jesse's favorite treat. One by one, we tested his reactions to the foods he ate; his regular supplements, including vitamin C, brewer's yeast, and a blend of omega oils marketed for dogs; and his shampoo. When the testing was done, a report was printed out showing the items that Jesse had reacted most strongly to. Brewer's yeast topped the list.

Some Good Things Aren't for Everyone

Some dogs' inability to handle brewer's yeast, a substance that most pets seem to take without a problem, shows that even though a supplement or remedy may be natural and widely accepted it doesn't mean it's right for every dog and cat. When looking for ways to support our pets, we must always remember that every animal is an individual with his own particular needs.

Brewer's yeast, a natural food additive, has become a popular alternative for discouraging fleas, replacing pesticide sprays or collars. Many animals can tolerate it well. But I've seen quite a few who cannot. Bioenergetic assessment indicated that Jesse could not handle brewer's yeast, and this probably explained his diarrhea and smelly ears. Animals who cannot tolerate brewer's yeast will likely develop signs of unwellness such as lethargy, diarrhea, and inflamed or infected ears, and these symptoms can become chronic. If they are not assessed holistically and the underlying stressor is not identified, they may be diagnosed with inflammatory bowel disease, develop an immune imbalance that evolves into an autoimmune condition, or suffer from nasty, stubborn ear problems. Further, if they are treated for their symptoms in a mainstream way, they may be given antibiotics, which will likely worsen the dysbiotic stress they are already experiencing. A holistic perspective tries to find the underlying cause of the problem and remove it, then support the living terrain with natural methods to help it return to homeostasis.

Jennifer was astonished to learn that Jesse had reacted negatively to brewer's yeast. Not only did she give it to him as a supplement, she discovered it was also an additive in his kibble. The lesson Jennifer learned from this experience is an important one—to always add a grain of salt when you read or hear claims that a product will be beneficial to your dog or cat's health. Not long after Jesse had been bioenergetically assessed, Jennifer called to tell me that she had removed all brewer's yeast from his diet and that his symptoms had cleared up entirely within a few days. Fortunately, we had caught the problem early, while Jesse's living terrain still had enough resilience to return itself to wellness without needing proactive support from us.

Jesse's greatest asset was having a human companion who knew that he needed help. This brings us to the important issue of when to bring your dog or cat to see the vet and how, from a holistic point of view, to prepare for the visit.

The Veterinary Coach and the Client-Collaborator

Generally speaking, people take their pets to see their vet for three reasons. One is because their dog or cat has been injured or shows signs of unwellness or illness. The second is because the pet needs a vaccination. And the third is in response to a reminder from their vet that their dog or cat is due for an annual checkup.

It goes without saying that both mainstream and holistic veterinarians would urge you to bring your pet to the vet for the first reason. However, because pharmaceutical companies have promoted the idea that a dog or cat needs to receive a booster vaccination each year, most vets who follow the mainstream medical approach have accepted this idea and have therefore combined the annual checkup visit with the vaccination visit. In the case of older pets, they may at the same time do standardized tests of the animal's vital organs, such as the kidney, liver, and heart.

Because I approach pet care from a holistic perspective, a vaccination schedule does not dictate the timing of my clients' visits as I do not recommend annual vaccinations for the dogs and cats I see. Nevertheless, primarily for preventive purposes, I recommend a vet visit at least once a year regardless of the state of your pet's health—even more often if your dog or cat is aging or prone to having problems. I use these visits to do an annual *wellness* assessment—including a clinical examination—and to take the opportunity to advise my clients about such things as heartworm, rabies, and any other concerns they may have.

Just as important, the annual visit gives my clients a chance to update me on the state of their pet's health so I can do my job as their veterinary coach. Sometimes, that means acknowledging clients for the obvious vitality, sheer joyfulness, and pleasure in life their pet exudes, or because a dog or cat was ill or unwell and is now showing signs of improvement. Sometimes it means suggesting activities and dietary changes to improve the animal's wellness or to support a pet whose living situation has changed or whose stage of life calls for it. And sometimes it means that I consult a qualified herbalist, chiropractor, acupuncturist, or bioenergetic tester for services that will add support for ongoing or recurring health conditions such as arthritis or allergies. On some occasions, of course, it means that I am able to catch a weakness in the pet's living terrain and intervene before it develops into something more serious.

For whatever reasons you visit your vet—at least once a year or when you notice signs and symptoms that don't seem right and you don't know what to do to clear them up on your own—*you need to be prepared.* Too often clients approach their vets as the source of all knowledge and insight about their dog or cat's health and consider their own experiences with their pet as having little or no value. Nothing could be further from the truth. Although you should expect your vet to have skills and information beyond what you expect of a layperson, you are the person who knows close at hand your dog or cat's daily habits and normal demeanor. You have much to contribute to the discussion of her state of health as well as to the healing plan your vet will develop. The following guidelines will help you get the most out of your visit.

Reassure Your Pet

Animals often become emotionally stressed out when taken to the vet. After all, once there, someone they may never have met before and who is not part of the family will handle them. They may also be upset about riding in the car if they aren't used to it. As well, some medical tests are uncomfortable or painful, and animals don't understand what it is all about. There are several steps you can take to make the appointment less difficult for your dog or cat.

For starters, calmly explain to him that you're going to see someone who will offer some help so that he can feel better. It doesn't matter whether he understands your words as long as he feels your love, reassurance, and good intentions. Assure him that he will be fine. Do this, but on the other hand don't make too big a deal out of it, lest he take it to mean that he *does* have reason to be anxious. Flower remedies can help soothe his fears and ease his stress. Give them as needed before you leave home, during the ride, possibly again at the clinic, and on the way home. (See Chapter 7.)

HOW TO PREPARE AHEAD OF TIME

Before your appointment, take note of the signs and symptoms that concern you, as Jennifer did for her dog Jesse. If you write them down, bring along your notes to help you remember everything you want to report. Be ready to describe signs of obvious illness; any *early signs of unwellness,* as described in Chapter 5, and whatever else you may have noticed from using your *six senses,* as described in Chapter 3.

If this is your dog or cat's first time seeing a particular vet, bring any records you may have of his previous veterinary history, or arrange to have them transferred from his previous veterinarian to the new one. Even if you can't locate all his records, do your best to report all the surgeries, vaccinations, drugs, and antibiotics he may have received in

While your dog or cat is being examined, stay nearby and watch for him to communicate with you. Don't ignore him. One reason animals get frightened at the vet's office may be because they are often handled as objects to be inspected, instead of as living beings who have their own integrity. If he looks at you questioningly, reassure him. Be calm yourself so he can take his cues from you. Because you are the person closest to him, he may look to you for clues about whether he is safe. You are probably his only familiar landmark in the place.

It is understandable that you may be anxious about your pet's health during the visit, but be aware that your anxiety may be contagious to your dog or cat, so do what you can to keep yourself on an even keel. If you breathe deeply and sigh occasionally, it may help to calm both of you. If you are concerned that you won't be as steady as you'd like to be, ask a calmer family member or friend whom your pet trusts to be with him during the physical part of the exam, instead of you.

---

the past, as well as the names of any drugs and supplements you currently give him. Also, be prepared to discuss his diet—*everything* he eats and drinks in the course of a normal day.

SHARE YOUR OBSERVATIONS WITH YOUR VET

Your veterinarian will need to know why you brought your dog or cat to the clinic and what you have observed about his health that concerns you. She'll probably start by asking you about his immediate problem, especially if he is in need of urgent help. Or, if this is the first time she has ever seen your pet or if she thinks holistically, she may want to find out about his long-term health and overall background before she asks about anything else. Don't just sit back and respond passively to your vet's questions. Be an active participant. If you think something you have noticed may be important, tell her about it whether she has asked you or not. *You make the judgement call* on whether your vet is picking up the information you think is significant.

As your vet attempts to figure out the cause of your pet's problem, remember that every health care professional is guided by a way of thinking. If she is thinking holistically, she will take into account the biggest possible picture. Or she may be thinking from the opposite—reductionist—perspective, trying to isolate a single cause for a problem while ruling out all other factors. Keep in mind that, as explained in Chapter 1, you may not be able to tell your vet's way of thinking based on the modalities she employs. In other words, some veterinarians who base their approach on mainstream modalities such as pharmaceutical drugs may also incorporate some holistic practices such as taking into account the cat or dog's emotional state, lifestyle, or physical environment. Other vets may follow mainstream goals such as focusing on getting rid of symptoms instead of looking deeper for their underlying cause, even though they may use natural modalities such as acupuncture and homeopathy. The more clearly you understand the differences between the two approaches, the better you will be able to tell whether *your* way of thinking is compatible with your vet's. This will give you the basis for clearer communication. Regardless of her primary approach, if your veterinarian is open-minded, you'll find it easier to discuss a variety of possible causes and solutions for your dog or cat's trouble. But if she isn't open-minded and you think she isn't sufficiently taking into account an observation you believe is important, you will need to decide whether to move on to somebody else.

REVIEW YOUR PET'S LIFE HISTORY

When a client brings a dog or a cat to my clinic for the first time, I prefer to learn the animal's life history before I find out anything else. This is important not only for a younger animal but also for a mature one. Whether a pet is two, twelve, or twenty years old, knowing the life history will help a holistic vet view the current problem in the broadest possible context as he looks for the sources of stress that are causing it.

To be an effective collaborator with your vet, rehearse your pet's history ahead of time. Think back to when you first got him. How long has he been with you? Did you adopt him when he was a kitten or a puppy, or was he already an adult? Did you get him from a breeder? Or did he come from a puppy or kitten mill or from a pet store that gets the animals it sells from puppy or kitten mills? Did you adopt him from a shelter or rescue group, from an ad in the paper, or from a friend? Or was he feral when you brought him under your wing? This kind of information will prompt a holistic vet to consider whether genetic stress or stress related to your pet's early development may underlie the present problem.

Review your dog or cat's long-term social and emotional experience. If his first home was not with you, how many homes did he have before he came to you? Was he kept indoors or outdoors most of the time? Was he tied up or confined in a pen, or did he roam at large? Has he ever been neglected or abused either physically or emotionally, or do you suspect that he has? Physical abuse can include everything from overly harsh treatment to outright violence to deprivation of basic survival needs such as food and water. Social and emotional neglect can include denying an animal opportunities to play and have contact with his own kind and others, especially while he's growing up, and prolonged periods with little or no social contact, as many backyard dogs experience who are tied up outside all the time. A cat left alone in a house for more than a couple of days while his people vacation abroad and who sees only the neighbor who comes in to feed him once a day is another example of social and emotional neglect.

Also be ready to provide the details of your pet's long-term physical health. What significant illnesses or injuries has he suffered over the course of his life? Does he have an illness that returns time and again? For example, has your dog had chronic, off-and-on diarrhea since he was a puppy, or does your cat develop frequent upper respiratory infections? Be sure to report what types of vaccinations your pet has received throughout his life and how often they have been repeated. Also inform your vet about every surgery your dog or cat has had, and the age they were performed. Has he had any dental work done? Was he ever put on any antibiotics, steroids, or other pharmaceutical drugs in the past? And finally, has he always shone with wellness, or never fully blossomed?

The history of an animal's diet, from birth up to the present, supplies crucial information to the holistic vet. Let her know whether your pet has been fed processed or unprocessed foods during various periods of his life and, if possible, give the brand names. You may be lucky enough to know what his mother was fed while he was in the womb. Was he weaned onto processed or unprocessed food? Give a clear outline of the kinds of food he has eaten up to the present time, including supplements you may give him. Don't forget to include the kinds of treats he has been given—treats make up a surprising proportion of the modern pet's diet.

If your vet doesn't ask about your dog or cat's life history, offer to tell her anyway. If she doesn't want to hear about it or says it's not important, this is a clue that she is not a holistic thinker. If you suspect this is the case, be aware that her narrow focus will reflect in both her diagnosis of your pet's problem and the treatment she recommends. If you are not satisfied with her approach, get a second opinion.

THE REASON YOU CAME IN

When you tell your veterinarian why you brought your dog or cat to the clinic, describe not only any obvious signs of illness, but also the subtle signs of unwellness. Be as clear and specific as you can. Be sure to include how you perceive your pet to be feeling emotionally. Don't

Let Your Vet Know How to Relate to Your Pet

Your veterinarian will probably start the physical examination while you are discussing your pet's history. Remember that you know your pet best, and if you can think of less upsetting ways to approach and handle him, don't hesitate to say so. Say a bit about his nature—whether he's fearful, had once been abused, or has strong protective tendencies. For example, if your cat is afraid to be picked up, let your vet know that so she can approach gently. If your dog is the type who takes a direct stare as a challenge, tell her not to look him in the eye. Not only will your guidance make the experience easier for the animal, but it might also help prevent the vet and her staff from being bitten or scratched.

leave out what you sense about his health status even if you can't pin it to a precise symptom.

Tell your vet about any recent events that led up to any problems at hand. For example, if your pet is limping and in pain and you know that this started right after he chased a squirrel around a tree, say so. Or, if his symptoms began soon after you gave him his daily dose of medication, report that. Did you notice any other signs or symptoms in recent weeks or months? Mention them even if they seem unrelated to his current problem.

Be sure to include your pet's present life circumstances. Is he on antibiotics, steroids, painkillers, or other pharmaceuticals? Has he had any vaccinations recently? Does he have any known sensitivities to foods or allergens of any kind? Does he have a quiet life at home? Do you have children or other pets? Finally, bring up any important changes that have taken place in his life recently, such as a new pet being added to the household, a new baby, a change in your schedule, or moving to a new house. Remember that an animal's wellness will be affected by any strains or tension between family members; mention at least briefly whether your household has any of these kinds of problems, because they can provide important clues about what your pet may be coping with.

WEEKEND WARRIOR HEALTH PROBLEMS

A pet's lifestyle can provide the key to why a particular health issue has emerged, especially when the issue would not be expected for his age or breed. These days, I'm seeing a lot of younger dogs with problems that used to be the domain of older, fatter dogs. For instance Espresso, a four-year-old chocolate Labrador retriever, suddenly went lame and broke a ligament in his left knee. The injury was surgically repaired. Three years later, when his left hock became swollen and sore, his people brought him to my clinic for a second perspective. We X-rayed him and found severe arthritis in both hocks, in the stifle joint that had been repaired, and in several other joints as well.

I was perplexed. A dog from an athletic breed, such as a Lab, should not suffer a spontaneous cruciate ligament break at four years old nor have arthritic changes in his joints by age seven. Espresso's history suggested that he had always had weak joints, which to my view must have been induced by underlying, metabolic problems. As well, Espresso was probably a weekend warrior—the term I use for a dog who sits around all week and then is taken out on weekends to run. The lack of conditioning combined with sudden, intense exercise could have led him to break that ligament simply by twisting it.

To help Espresso maintain reasonable mobility and quality of life in spite of the degenerative changes that had occurred, we set him up for physiotherapy, veterinary orthopedic manipulation (VOM), a weekly swim in a hydrotherapy pool at a nearby dog spa, joint-easy exercise to help his body keep some overall tone, plus nutritional support. In a case like this, I would not expect the arthritis itself to disappear, but I am always hopeful.

We are seeing a tremendous increase of ruptured cruciates and similar problems in dogs too young to be experiencing these issues. I believe several factors probably combine to cause this: genetically inherited weakness, less than optimal nutrition, and exercise that is too intense for the animal's degree of fitness. It's frustrating to see these injuries happening to athletic breeds when they can be prevented with appropriate exercise, nutritional changes, and better breeding practices.

The Four Fields of Tests

Once your vet has obtained as much information as possible from your report, she has available four fields of scientific tests that can provide more information about a pet's health status and help her clarify some possibilities about what the problem is.

The physical field. In these tests, the vet observes the physical signs of illness, including gait, general movement, and the condition of the eyes, skin, gums, and so on. She will check for lumps and bumps, listen to the animal's heart, look into his ears, and note whether he has painful and tender areas in response to her touch. Don't hesitate to draw her attention to the areas you want her to examine.

The biochemical field. This field of tests examines the living terrain's natural biochemistry by sampling and measuring body fluids. Blood tests and urinalysis are two useful and familiar examples of this field. Other biochemical tests look at joint fluid, cerebrospinal fluid, and so on.

The imaging field. This field includes all the tests that capture and examine images of the body. X-rays, ultrasound, computerized tomography (CT) scans, and magnetic resonance imaging (MRI) are common examples.

The bioenergetic assessment field. These tests measure subtle shifts in the living terrain's bioenergetic field. Its most well-known tools are muscle testing, computerized electrodermal screening (EDS), and auricular medicine testing, among others.

Caleb's Mystery Illness

Caleb, a lively Bouvier des Flandres dog, went off his food one day. He seemed depressed, was warm to the touch, and had several bouts of diarrhea. By midnight, his worsening signs of unwellness worried Susan enough to prompt her to make an emergency call to her rural mainstream veterinarian, who agreed to meet them at the clinic as soon as they could get there. In the wee hours of the morning, Susan sat with her dog as he lay resting on the floor of the clinic while the vet examined him.

Caleb was running a low fever, but a physical exam revealed no other signs of illness. The vet suggested that blood tests might offer more clues to what was wrong, and Susan agreed to have them done. After the vet drew a vial of blood from Caleb's leg, Susan took him home again and waited for the results.

The next day the vet called to report that the tests showed a strange pattern in Caleb's blood work—his platelet count was abnormally high. However, this information alone was inconclusive, and all the signs put together did not fit a clear diagnostic picture. Because the vet was concerned that Caleb might have a serious condition, she said that further biochemical tests might be helpful; even so, there was no guarantee that they would clarify his situation.

STANDARD TESTS ARE DAMAGE REPORTS

Three fields of assessment are standard medical tests—physical, biochemical, and imaging—and are used by both holistic and mainstream vets. Holistic vets may use the fourth field, bioenergetic assessment, in addition to the other kinds. The first three fields primarily indicate degenerative changes that have already resulted from other, underlying problems. In other words, standard tests are damage reports. As a rule, they cannot detect the signs of unwellness that warn us that a full-blown illness may be coming down the pike. On the upside, they let us know what damage has been done. On the downside, the information they

Susan was grateful for the vet's responsiveness and her honesty about the limits of the methods she had available to assess Caleb's problem. She tried to figure out the most balanced road to take. Doing more tests would mean putting him through the stress of another trip to the clinic and having blood drawn again. It would also be costly; the first round of blood work had already cost $300 and hadn't helped solve the problem. And by then, Caleb seemed to be rallying on his own. Susan and the vet agreed not to go ahead with further tests as long as Caleb continued to improve.

Caleb recovered from his mystery illness and appeared to be fine for a while. The next time his blood work was checked, his platelets were back to normal. But because mainstream medicine monitors illness rather than wellness, the underlying unwellness that made him susceptible to illness was not identified. A few months later, he became gravely ill with canine distemper. (See Chapter 7 to find out how remedies that support the living terrain saved Caleb's life, beginning on page 157.)

provide is tantamount to telling us that the horse has already escaped from the barn and it's too late to stop it.

Because mainstream veterinary medicine relies on standard tests alone, it has fewer tools than a broader, holistic approach can offer for assessing a pet's health. Nevertheless, standard tests can be very useful and have a place in holistic practice. But you should also be aware that sometimes they may waste time and money because they cannot detect and analyze unwellness.

I'm not recommending that standard tests should be avoided, because they can be valuable in diagnosing disease. If Caleb's blood work had revealed a diagnosable condition, it would have been better for Susan and the vet to know this so they could try to help him. But as a rule, the first three fields of tests cannot detect the unwellness that makes an animal susceptible to illness. This means that the kind of results they produce don't help us predict illness. And, because the damage that standard tests can detect is already done, veterinarians who rely solely on these kinds of assessments find themselves doing damage control rather than focusing on prevention. We must be realistic about what tests can and cannot do. This is why I have become a fan of bioenergetic assessment.

The Beauty of Bioenergetic Assessment

When a pet is not well, bioenergetic assessment—which holistic health care professionals sometimes refer to as *energy testing*—can give us more information about his condition than standard tests can yield. As I described in Chapter 1, an animal's body, or living terrain, consists of tissues, organs, glands, hormones, and other structures and systems. Tissues, organs, and fluids consist of cells; those cells, in turn, are bits and pieces of energy. Energy both forms and flows through the body. Bioenergetic assessment builds on the assumption that changes can be discerned in living energy before illness occurs.[1] Consequently, measuring these changes can be a great diagnostic tool for helping our dogs and cats return to homeostasis. This is the beauty of bioenergetic assessment.

Bioenergetic assessment offers three major advantages over standard tests:

First, it detects changes in the energy field, drawing our attention to a state of unwellness of which we may otherwise have been unaware and leading us to investigate subtler aspects of the animal's health.

Second, by identifying unwellness before it manifests into physical illness, it gives us the opportunity to prevent tissue damage that could lead to illness.

The History of Bioenergetic Assessment

The idea that life force energy flows through every being is not new. It dates back in healing traditions for millennia. It can be found, for example, in the approaches of Ayurveda and traditional Chinese medicine, and among peoples of Africa and Hawaii, the aborigines of Australia, the Maori of New Zealand, across the Americas, in major world religions including Judeo-Christian traditions, and among healers and scientists throughout European history. Hippocrates, the founder of what has become mainstream medicine in the West, maintained that good health depends upon the free flow of this energy. Since early in the twentieth century, Western scientists have made discoveries in quantum physics that support the notion that there's a vital life force. Although they have developed ways to measure it, their research is not yet reflected in the practice of most mainstream doctors or veterinarians.

However, highly developed contemporary diagnostic technologies such as magnetic resonance imaging (MRI), electrocardiogram (EKG), electroencephalogram (EEG), and others are based on this concept and research.[2]

Finally, it gives us clues about where to look for the underlying stressor that's causing the pet's unwellness or illness.

DIFFERENT METHODS OF ENERGY TESTING

In bioenergetic assessment, ancient understandings and recent research come together in new tools that register imbalances in an animal's biomagnetic field and help us pinpoint the stressor that's causing his unwellness or illness. New methods emerge all the time: for example, some health care professionals use muscle testing, others use machines, and some measure the pet physically. Each approach has its merit. We'll look at three of these methods.

Each method offers not only diagnostic assistance but also help in determining which remedies might support that individual's return to homeostasis. Each one also provides a technique that can help to correct the energy imbalance that is causing the unwellness or illness. For the moment, we'll look solely at their diagnostic capabilities; in the next chapter we'll look at how they can aid healing.

Muscle testing is a technique derived from applied kinesiology, which is used for diagnosing both humans and animals. Applied kinesiology is based on the understanding that each muscle corresponds to a particular part of the body. If a muscle shows strength when tested in a special way, this indicates health in the body's corresponding organs; whereas if it shows weakness, this indicates a health problem in those organs.[3] This method does not test crude muscle strength, as a test in a gym might do; rather, it tests energy tracks that it accesses through muscle response.

Electrodermal screening (EDS) involves a device originally developed to measure electrical resistance at acupuncture points. An abnormal reading at a specific point indicates a problem in the corresponding organ or gland.[4] For years my clinic used computerized electrodermal screening—an EDS device hooked up to a computer that records the readings—with dogs and cats and had great success.

When assessing animals, both muscle testing and electrodermal screening use a person as a surrogate or vector to obtain the energy reading. For muscle testing, there are advantages to having a person trained in the technique to be the vector, because "reading" the response requires skill and experience.[5] In EDS, it is normal for the client to act as the surrogate. In either case, doing the test in a quiet, comfortable room is important to avoid distractions and sudden noises that might alarm the dog or cat. The precise technique varies for these two tests, but generally speaking, bottled or bagged substances are held by the surrogate or touched to the animal's body in such a way that the animal's energy response to the substance registers through the surrogate. In EDS, the response is recorded, in turn, on a computer. Both tests give us an excellent way to discover which foodstuffs, supplements, homeopathics, and sometimes herbals will be most helpful to this pet and which should be avoided.

Auricular medicine assessment measures changes in an individual's energy field through points in the external ear that are believed to correspond to organs, glands, and other parts of the body. As in muscle testing and EDS, auricular medicine assessment typically registers an animal's energy response to substances. Conductive filters are positioned on the animal, which are connected to metal plates on which test substances are placed. In this case, the test substances include organs and tissues, as well as foodstuffs and remedies. The results, as with the other forms of bioenergetic assessment, give us a picture of the pet's present state of health and help us determine what is blocking his living terrain from returning to homeostasis.[6] I currently use this method in my clinic.

I recognize that it can be hard to wrap our minds around the concept of energy flow and to take the notion further into accessing energy flow for diagnostic testing. And there are still a lot of unknowns in the field. But in my veterinary practice, I have experimented with a number of different diagnostic formats, including standard medical tests, muscle testing, EDS, and auricular medicine assessment, and I find the information that bioenenergetic assessment reveals to be invaluable. Energy medicine is based on quantum physics, which most of us don't understand. Most of us don't understand nuclear fission, either, but we do know that when we flip a switch an electric light will come on. We may not understand how an MRI works, but we know that it gets results. Like nuclear fission and MRIs, energy testing gets results. That's what's important when it comes to the health of our pets.

WHICH METHOD IS BEST?

When I started doing bioenergetic testing with my patients, I located a qualified energy medicine professional who brought her equipment to the clinic to assist us. In the early years, she used the EDS method, and later, for her own reasons, she switched to auricular medicine assessment. Because this is her speciality, we offer the technique she uses.

I don't recommend one method of bioenergetic assessment over another. We've had great success using both EDS and auricular medicine assessment. A veterinarian may be within your reach who can provide this service, as I am able to do. Each year, the number of veterinarians who follow a holistic approach is increasing, as is their use of bioenergetic assessment both for diagnosis and to develop healing plans. However, health care professionals who are qualified to use these techniques are still relatively rare in the United States and Canada, even though tens of thousands use them throughout the world. This is unfortunate, because I recommend that you work with only a qualified professional and only if she is working alongside, and under the guidance of, your veterinarian. Bioenergetic medicine is not a parlor trick, although some people may use it that way. It is serious stuff—it's medical diagnosis. There's a big difference between someone who uses these techniques for fun versus someone who uses them diagnostically every day of the week and in consultation with a qualified veterinarian. I find this approach to diagnosis to be so valuable that I look forward to the day when it is widely available.

The information gathering is complete after all the tests and the physical examination are done and you have shared your observations with your vet. When you and your vet are satisfied that the underlying cause of the problem has been determined, your vet will recommend a healing plan. What happens next will crucially depend on whether or not your vet's knowledge and experience is limited to mainstream approaches and modalities. Her knowledge and experience will determine how many tools she has available with which to address the problem.

ENDNOTES

1. Michael H. Cohen, "Energy Healing: An Emerging Enigma," in *Beyond Complementary Medicine: Legal and Ethical Perspectives on Health Care and Human Evolution* (Ann Arbor: University of Michigan Press, 2000), 181.

2. Kenneth S. Cohen, "Roots and Branches," in *The Way of Qigong, the Art and Science of Chinese Energy Healing* (New York: Ballantine Books, 1997), 23–27; Larry Trivieri Jr. and John W. Anderson, eds., "Energy Medicine," in *Alternative Medicine: The Definitive Guide,* 2nd ed. (Berkeley/Toronto: Celestial Arts, 2002), 201–202.

3. Larry Trivieri Jr. and John W. Anderson, eds., "Applied Kinesiology," in *Alternative Medicine: The Definitive Guide,* 2nd ed. (Berkeley/Toronto: Celestial Arts, 2002), 71–75.

4. For background on EDS, see Larry Trivieri Jr. and John W. Anderson, eds., "Energy Medicine," in *Alternative Medicine: The Definitive Guide,* 2nd ed. (Berkeley/Toronto: Celestial Arts, 2002), 206–207.

5. Wendy Volhard and Kerry Brown, "Kinesiology," in *Holistic Guide for a Healthy Dog,* 2nd ed. (New York: Howell Books, 2004), 163-66.

6. Extensive information on auricular medicine is in Bryan L. Frank, MD, and Nader E. Solima, MD, "Introduction to Auricular Medicine," in *Auricular Therapy: A Comprehensive Text* (Bloomington, IN: AuthorHouse Press, 2006), chapter 17. Also see the website of Cherri Campbell, DiHom, "Inner Health: Auricular Medicine and Homeopathy," www.innerhealth.ca/cherri.html (accessed February 5, 2009).

PART FOUR

The Secret to Healing

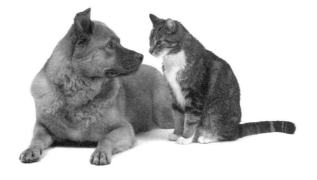

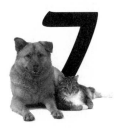

Choosing Therapies to Restore Wellness

Susan and Caleb, her Bouvier des Flandres dog, had just returned from a fifteen-hundred-mile (twenty-four-hundred kilometer) car trip when she called our clinic to say that the three-year-old dog had distemper. Two weeks earlier, Caleb had experienced a day or two of vomiting and projectile, foul-smelling diarrhea, but he seemed to recover, so they headed off on schedule to visit Susan's friend in rural Iowa. Once there, Caleb began to lose interest in his food. A couple of days before they left for home, he became quiet and his eyes began to trickle greenish goo. Susan sought a local vet's advice. Two days and nights of traveling lay ahead of them. Should she bring him in to be checked out or head home to her own vet and hope he didn't take a turn for the worse along the way? Neither Susan nor the vet she consulted suspected anything as serious as distemper—Caleb's signs were nonspecific and he did not seem to be urgently ill. So the vet advised Susan to head for home and seek help from her own veterinarian.

Soon after they hit the road, Caleb developed a mucusy cough and his nose dripped clear fluid; his breath and body odor became strangely offensive. Having successfully used homeopathy for herself for decades,

Susan knew of a remedy that matched Caleb's upper respiratory symptoms and his demeanor, so she picked some up in the first major town they passed through. The next morning, his cough was completely gone and his eyes were clear once again. But over the course of the day, his diarrhea and vomiting became significantly worse. In the evening, he vomited yellow bile containing tiny flecks of blood. Fortunately, his symptoms did not worsen dramatically while they slept and in the morning, they got back on the road.

Once they arrived home, with my clinic yet a further eighty miles away, Susan rushed Caleb to her local animal hospital for an assessment. Although his temperature had now reached 103.6°F (39.7°C), his symptoms did not yet suggest a definite diagnosis. The vet drew blood for tests and Susan took the dog home again.

That night the Bouvier's breathing became loud and congested as though he were snoring while awake and by morning, creamy yellow liquid gushed out of his nostrils. This clue made the difference—it enabled Susan to realize that Caleb fit the picture for canine distemper. Because she had made a personal choice not to have him immunized against the disease, she had kept herself well informed of its signs and symptoms so she would be prepared to recognize it.

With the quality of his nasal discharge, a fever of 104°F (40°C), and a red measles-like rash developing on his abdomen, the local vet had enough evidence to confirm that Caleb had the classic signs of canine distemper virus (CDV). But she also admitted that mainstream veterinary medicine could not cure this very serious illness. It could only offer treatments to minimize the symptoms, such as IV fluids to prevent dehydration and antibiotics to avoid complications such as pneumonia or conjunctivitis, and hope that the virus would run its course. But dogs often die of CDV and the few survivors sustain neurological damage so frequently that many vets now recommend euthanizing distemper patients rather than allowing them to suffer.

Undaunted by this grave prognosis, Susan decided to seek a different approach. She had read previously that holistic veterinarians had facilitated hundreds of successful recoveries from CDV with the aid of natural therapies that support the immune system[1]. Based on her experience, her confidence was strongest in homeopathy.

She called my clinic for guidance about which remedy to use and at which strength. Following homeopathic practice, we matched Caleb's symptoms to Distemperinum—a homeopathic remedy made from discharges of CDV-infected dogs. We recommended that she begin with a fairly low potency to see if it would prompt him enough to heal without overwhelming him. If it didn't, she could increase the potency. (See pages 164–165 for more on homeopathic remedies.)

Less than a half hour after giving Caleb his first dose, his temperature dropped to 102.4°F (39.1°C). Susan dosed him twice more that night and also trickled down his throat a gentle form of vitamin C dissolved in a little water to give him supplementary support.[2] She had available cool chicken broth and a little water with honey for him to drink when he was ready.

The next morning, Caleb's temperature was steady at 102.4°F (39.1°C) and his nasal discharge was much looser. After another dose of homeopathic Distemperinum, Caleb started asking for food and was given a tiny natural biscuit or two to munch so as not to aggravate his stressed digestive system.

The third morning after he'd started on homeopathy, his temperature was down to 101.8°F (38.6°C). Susan added slippery elm to his chicken broth to soothe his ravaged gastrointestinal tract. His nasal discharge became clear and colorless once again. On the fourth day of receiving homeopathic support, Caleb's breathing was silent and easy again, his measles rash was fading, and his sweet breath was returning. His temperature was still dropping, so Susan began reintroducing him to his usual unprocessed diet, carefully adding a little raw meat to his cooked mashed vegetables. By the fifth day his temperature was normal for a dog, at 100.2°F (37.9°C). By the eighth day, the distemper symptoms were completely gone and he was back on his full diet. Caleb never developed the neurological damage that survivors of distemper so often incur.

Caleb's story is a prime example of how remedies that support the immune system—those that are commonly associated with the holistic approach—can help an animal recover from even a deadly virus that mainstream medicine cannot cure. But the correct remedy alone did not save Caleb's life. There's no question in my mind that his person's holistic approach to his health care and her commitment to nursing him through his illness are what made the difference. She took responsibility for the decisions she made about immunization and kept herself well informed. She fed him a diet of unprocessed foods, which maximized the potential of his living terrain to respond positively to a supportive therapy. She made sure he was given exactly the kind of medicine needed to motivate his immune system to overcome the threat of a very dangerous stressor. All of these were crucial to his triumph over a devastating illness.

Caleb's story also demonstrates that the holistic way relies on more than its remedies. As I explained in Chapter 1, virtually any remedy can serve the goals of either the holistic way or mainstream medicine. In addition to selecting the most helpful remedies, the holistic approach looks for the hidden stress factors that led to the situation, adjusts the animal's diet to better support her living terrain, and modifies her environment to meet her needs. As well, the holistic way favors therapies that work with life's flow rather than those that work against it, because they, like the holistic philosophy, are based on the premise that **the secret of healing is to respectfully motivate the living terrain to heal itself.**

Nevertheless, at times circumstances may call for modalities that interfere with, rather than support, the living terrain. In my view, part

A Word about Terms

When discussing modalities, I try not use terms such as Western, Eastern, complementary, alternative, and so on, because I find these terms problematic. For example, mainstream medicine is often referred to as Western. But homeopathy, which was discovered in Germany, is also Western—and it has made major contributions to the development of holistic theory and practice. Further, modalities such as acupuncture that came from the East may take on altered forms when imported into a Western context. None of these terms sufficiently take into account methods arising from continents such as Africa or Australia. And to me, each of the terms *complementary, alternative,* and *conventional* reflects in its own way the status quo of the twentieth century, in which the mainstream approach has been widely viewed as the enlightened form of health care and any other approach has been seen as deviant from it. I believe it is more useful to discuss modalities in terms of how they affect the living terrain.[3]

of being holistic is to keep an open mind. By assessing each patient as an individual and remembering that every problem is born of its own peculiar circumstances, we can choose the therapies most suitable for the situation. To understand which therapies will optimally meet a pet's needs, it's important to understand some crucial differences between them.

Choose Therapies for Their Differences

Every health care therapy affects the living terrain at a physical, a biochemical, or an energetic level, and some affect more than one level. Physical modalities, such as chiropractic and massage, act upon the living terrain's manifested form. Biochemical modalities, such as botanicals and low-potency homeopathics, work on its underlying bio-chemistry. Energetic modalities, such as acupuncture, flower essences, and high-potency homeopathics, act upon deeper substrata, the body's energy fields.

Modalities also differ in whether they support the living terrain's ability to heal itself or invade it and impose their order upon it. The great majority of healing modalities support the living terrain. In agreement with holistic principles, these therapies release blocked energy that prevents the body from reaching homeostasis. However, they must be used as part of a multifaceted holistic approach that includes finding and addressing the causes of stress. When used primarily to eliminate troublesome symptoms—a mainstream goal—supportive remedies will not bring about long-term recovery as they are designed to do, and the pet may have a relapse.

In contrast with modalities that respect the body, surgery, pharmaceuticals, and radiation invade the living terrain and force a different way of being upon it. They are familiar to most of us because such modalities became predominant in the twentieth century for complicated economic, political, and cultural reasons. They are based on the assumption that when the living terrain is not performing the way we would wish, it is appropriate to interfere with it. As a result of their aggressive action, they often cause iatrogenic stress. (See pages 81–84.) As Chapter 1 pointed out, they can save lives in certain situations and offer relief from pain. But I cannot emphasize enough that invasive modalities should only be used when they serve holistic goals—for example, to stabilize life after serious accidents, remove rapidly growing cancers to give supportive therapies a chance to work, reconstruct broken bones and ruptured tissue so they can heal, and ease the stress of acute and intolerable suffering. A good rule to follow is that remedies should always be the most effective possible while being the least invasive.

No matter which kind of therapy you may employ for your pet, I urge you to seek professional advice to ensure that you have selected an appropriate method and are using it properly. (See the Selected Resources in the Appendix.) The veterinarian should have qualifications for using the modality and experience administering it. Supportive remedies do not, as a rule, carry the dangers that mainstream therapies carry, and many of them can be bought in health food stores. But the fact that they may be easy to buy does not mean that they are unsophisticated and easy to use correctly, or that they will work for everybody. There is no recipe for healing that works for everybody. Besides, like so many things of true value, healing can't simply be bought. To be successful using any modality, you must understand the dynamics of how it works. Healing and health care are not a game; they take patience and commitment and require you to become intimately involved with the well-being of your pet.

A Repertoire of Useful Therapies

I appreciate being a holistic veterinarian especially when it comes to therapy. Whereas my mainstream colleagues tend to paint their picture of health in black and white, I have a full palette of colors available to me for designing healing plans for my clients' pets.

As each year passes, the number of modalities available that support the living terrain grows and their applications become more and more refined. Although I try to keep abreast of new approaches to therapy, I believe that my clinic offers greater benefit for the dogs and cats we see by selecting particular modalities, building up our knowledge of them, and gaining experience with using them. There are many other therapies available, but my clinic hasn't had a lot of experience with them. Therefore, the modalities I discuss below do not represent all the possibilities, nor do I mean to suggest that they are the best. Rather, I offer them as examples to compare the different actions of different therapies in light of what this book is about.

ACUPUNCTURE AND ACUPRESSURE

Acupuncture and acupressure have been used for many centuries. For example, they are key components of the ancient arts of traditional Chinese medicine (TCM) and Ayurvedic medicine. We use them in the clinic for a variety of purposes, among them as part of the NAET®4 approach to resolving allergies. Generally speaking, they stimulate energy tracts in the meridians of the body and thus motivate changes in the living terrain in its quest for homeostasis.

HOMEOPATHY

For more than two hundred years, homeopathic remedies—natural substances reduced to a highly diluted form through an involved process—have been used to energetically motivate the living terrain to return to homeostasis after stressors have pushed it out of balance. There are many types of homeopathic remedies, and their healing action varies depending on the substances on which they are based, the dilution of those substances, and the processes that are used to make them. Specific types of homeopathic remedies have either an energetic or a biochemical primary function, and in some cases they have both. The biochemical action of homeopathic remedies, however, is not equal to the biochemical action of other modalities, such as botanicals, nutraceuticals, and pharmaceuticals. These latter modalities add significant amounts of chemical or mineral substance to the living terrain, whereas homeopathic remedies add very minute traces of the substance, if any at all.

In choosing the correct remedy or combination remedy, the homeopath matches the action of particular remedies to the symptoms of the individual to rectify imbalances in the living terrain. The **single remedies** used in classical homeopathy have the highest dilutions, which, in homeopathic terms, means they have the greatest potency. Their action takes place solely at an energetic level because they are so highly diluted that they do not contain physical traces of the original substance. For consistent results, they need to be administered by an experienced and classically trained homeopath. **Complex remedies,** on the other hand, combine several remedies that have low dilutions. They are low-potency remedies whose action is not only energetic but also biochemical because they do contain minute physical traces of the original substance. I personally favor the use of complex remedies for pets because the single remedy approach of classical homeopathy requires the patient to describe the details of her symptoms in words, which animals cannot give us.

I also use several homeopathic remedies that are *primarily* biochemical in their action. **Gemmotherapy** uses remedies made from buds and young growing plants; **Schuessler tissue salts**, low-potency dilutions, help correct cellular deficiencies and support, detoxify, and rebuild the living terrain; and **Oligotherapy**, based on trace minerals in a highly diluted yet active form, helps correct functional disturbances by acting on the enzyme systems that are essential for normal metabolic function. By clearing the living terrain of toxins, these remedies unblock pathways so that the pet's vital energy can flow freely, which is necessary for wellness.

Homeopathic remedies can be obtained without prescription from homeopathic suppliers, health food stores, and some drugstores. Compared to most pharmaceuticals, they are inexpensive. However, using these remedies effectively requires a complex and sophisticated understanding. Although they are usually safe, they will be of limited value if not used under the direction of a qualified professional who is knowledgeable about homeopathics and experienced in using them.

BOTANICALS

Medicinal herbs have been used by healers and in medical practice from ancient times, and they are just as important to holistic care today. Eastern herbs are important components of traditional Chinese medicine (TCM) and Ayurvedic medicine, whereas Western herbs come from Europe and the First Nations peoples of the Americas. Usually used in combinations of several herbs together, they offer a multitude of options for supporting a living terrain that has lost homeostasis. Their biochemical action supports positive changes in the body's metabolism and encourages the drainage of toxins.

Aromatherapy uses the medicinal properties of the oils of various plants to both biochemically and energetically support the living terrain. They can be absorbed orally or through diffusers. We also use numerous **flower essences**, such as the Bach flower remedies, that offer gentle support for emotional stress through their energetic action. Our patients usually take them orally, but they, too, can be absorbed through a diffuser or even applied topically.

THERAPEUTIC NUTRITION

Nutrition is the keystone for maintaining wellness. Under normal circumstances, a well-balanced basic diet will provide the appropriate range and quantity of nutrients for a healthy living terrain. But when the body is under stress, supplementation may be necessary. Therapeutic nutritional supplements should synergize with any other healing modalities that are being used. In other words, the combination of modalities should produce effects that are greater than each modality would have on its own.

At my clinic, we use a range of **vitamins, minerals, amino acids, natural antioxidants, enzymes, and coenzyme** supplements to support a stressed living terrain. **Organotherapy** uses organ materials to supplement the specific organs that are under stress. Omega-rich plant, vegetable, fish, and other oils offer support to a disturbed immune system, improve the integrity of stressed joints, and bolster the condition of the skin and hair. **Probiotics**, which help correct dysbiotic stress, play a major role in healing because healthy digestion is crucial to proper immune system functioning and the general well-being of the living terrain.

CHIROPRACTIC THERAPY AND VETERINARY ORTHOPEDIC MANIPULATION (VOM)

Chiropractic therapy works on the physical level by helping restore the integrity of the spine and nervous system, both of which are essential to the health of the living terrain. Manually resolving subluxations in the spine can enormously benefit the living terrain by alleviating physical stress and helping the body reestablish homeostasis. **Veterinary orthopedic manipulation** (VOM) has similar goals to chiropractic, also working at a physical level to manually relieve stressed areas of the body. **Laser light therapy** acts on the physical level to stimulate tissue repair, helping reduce inflammation and restore homeostasis to localized areas of the living terrain.

PHYSICAL THERAPY

My clinic draws on services available at a rehabilitation facility to provide physical therapies that will support animals who are recovering from surgery or an illness. These services include **hydrotherapy**, which uses underwater treadmill systems, **therapeutic ultrasound**, and **muscular electrostimulation**, all of which support the living terrain both locally and systemically.

Massage provides physical benefits by helping relieve tight muscles and stimulate circulation in stressed areas of the body. It also has the advantage of being adaptable to home use and can greatly reinforce the bond between the cat or dog and her human companion. (See Dr. Michael W. Fox's books on healing touch in the Selected Bibliography in the Appendix.)

Tellington TTouch® and **Reiki** are examples of hands-on touch therapies that work on both the physical and the energetic levels to support the living terrain to return to homeostasis. When they are done by a person who is skilled and experienced in these healing arts, they accomplish their goals in a way that is very pleasurable to the cat or dog.

SURGERY

Surgery is a physical modality that forcibly reconfigures the living terrain. It is a drastic intervention that can repair structural damage that the living terrain cannot repair on its own. It can also remove severely diseased tissues, such as decaying teeth or clumps of cells that are dividing out of control (cancer), which, if left in the body, might kill or compromise the patient before a more supportive therapy has time to solve the problem. I regard surgery as primarily an emergency measure. Whenever I use it, I also employ other modalities such as homeopathic remedies, drainage complexes, flower remedies, massage, and others, both to support the living terrain as it heals and for the pet's longer-term wellness.

COLOR AND SOUND THERAPIES

As Temple Grandin has taught us so well, animals are in many ways more perceptive of their environment than are their human companions. (See Temple Grandin's books listed in the Selected Bibliography in the Appendix.) They are highly sensitive to color—they recognize color in spite of some common beliefs that they don't—and cats and dogs hear sounds at a wider range of frequencies and at lower volumes than humans hear them. As described in Chapter 3, their sensitivity to sight and sound can introduce sources of stress. However, we can use color and sound as therapeutic tools to relieve stress and support the return to homeostasis. We have much more to learn about these modalities.

PHARMACEUTICALS

Over the past century, the pharmaceutical industry has introduced thousands of drugs to address thousands of conditions. Both the number of drugs as well as the conditions are escalating. The goal of drug therapy is to dramatically and effectively counteract symptoms and modify metabolism. Drugs are valuable—under some circumstances, lifesaving—but they can also be detrimental because they invade and

Be Wary about Pharmaceuticals

When pharmaceuticals are recommended for your pet, be sure to investigate every aspect of the drug being prescribed. Ask your vet why it is being prescribed and about any abnormal reactions that may accompany its use. Ask whether there are less invasive approaches to achieve the desired effects and whether your cat or dog needs the medication. Ask what would happen if she is not given it. Your pet's wellness is at stake, so don't hesitate to be proactive and use your own good sense about using any drug.

disrupt the living terrain. They are biochemical in their action, but unlike the subtle biochemical action of low-potency homeopathic remedies, they introduce significant amounts of chemicals into the living terrain, either to make up for a shortfall in the natural occurrence of the chemical or to boost the amount of chemical naturally present.

Nutraceuticals and herbs also introduce significant amounts of chemicals for these same purposes, but they do so in a way that supports the normal workings of the living terrain. Pharmaceuticals, however, are designed to interfere with normal biochemical reactions and to impose a different balance in the living terrain, thus forcing it toward a particular outcome. By their very nature, they create stress on the living terrain and disturb homeostasis. The Food and Drug Administration of the United States and Health Canada's reports on abnormal reactions to nearly every drug used in veterinary medicine are frightening. (See the Selected Bibliography in the Appendix.)

In light of all of this, I use pharmaceuticals in emergencies when I believe that their action is called for, but I typically minimize the length of time they are used and employ them in combination with supportive remedies in certain conditions that appear to benefit from pharmaceutical intervention. I also search for less invasive methods to achieve the desired results.

A Holistic Perspective on Discomfort

When a woman named Meena's own health was seriously compromised and she could no longer look after her briard, she found a new home for him with people who followed the holistic way. After Buddy had been at his new home for a few months, Meena went to visit him. At the time, one of his ears was somewhat itchy and sore, and it smelled unpleasant. Buddy had long suffered from ear infections and Meena's vet had routinely prescribed antibiotics for them, but they kept coming back. Meena could see that Buddy had one of his infections now.

Thinking that his new people might not realize his ear needed attention, Meena mentioned it. They nodded casually and said they knew about it and were looking after it. The way they reacted perplexed her. Meena believed that an ear-infected dog should be rushed to the vet to receive drugs to treat the symptom; not to do so was tantamount to neglect. She did not understand that Buddy's new people saw his infection in a quite different light than she did. Instead of panicking, they had put him on a diet of unprocessed foods and were working with me in the long term to bring about a shift in his underlying condition so that he would not manifest ear infections as badly or as often in the future. We started him on homeopathic drainage remedies to help him flush out accumulated toxins. I also assessed that Buddy had a lot of resilience and I did not think his ear was seriously compromised, so instead of prescribing antibiotics I provided a mild ear wash that would help his ear restore the natural flora that it should normally contain. In holistic terms, the discharge from his ear was a positive sign that he was on the way to making that shift, and we did not intend to suppress his immune system's effort to clear itself.

Buddy's story illustrates a key difference between mainstream thinking and the holistic way. Both approaches take an uncomfortable symptom as an indication that something is wrong. But the holistic way views it as a signpost providing a clue to an underlying problem, and also as an

A Depressing Trend

Sadly, there is a growing trend to give antidepressant drugs such as clomipramine hydrochloride to pets to manage their behavioral problems. These drugs invade the highest level of the terrain—the brain—and cause biochemical changes to take place within it. We have no way of understanding their ramifications because we cannot communicate verbally with our pets. My advice is to avoid these drugs. When an animal behaves undesirably, try to find out why and look for ways to rectify the problem itself, instead of masking it. Many better methods are available for addressing behavioral issues, including modifying the animal's environment, giving them flower remedies to calm their energy, and positive training.

indication that the immune system is active and functioning. In holistic thinking, immune response is to be encouraged, not suppressed. When discomfort is too great we do seek to relieve it, but we do not want to stop it altogether because it gives us useful information. While working on deeper issues, we often tolerate and live with a certain amount of discomfort until true recovery happens or we determine that a pet cannot recover on its own and will need ongoing support. On the other hand, mainstream medicine views discomfort expressed by the body as unacceptable and something that should be relieved effectively and immediately. However, as a rule, and with some exceptions, it does not regard discomfort caused by its methods to be equally unacceptable.

The Four Modes of Stress Response

I as explained in Chapter 2, each pet will respond differently to stressors that challenge her living terrain. In a similar way, each pet will respond differently to the supportive therapies we use to stimulate her innate capacity to return to homeostasis. Some individuals have an energy reserve that allows them to respond well and recover quickly, whereas others don't have that reserve or ability to react. Consequently, when I am working out a plan to support the living terrain of a stressed-out pet, one of the most important factors I take into account is the dog or cat's ability to respond to the stress that the therapy will introduce.[5]

I refer to this ability to respond to stress as **the four modes of stress response.** Originally, the four modes were part of the basic theory of homeopathy[6], but I have further developed them to serve as a guide to how much therapeutic stress an individual animal can handle. Because you are your pet's primary caregiver—the one who knows her best, sees her every day, and most often administers her remedies—you will find it useful to understand how the four modes of stress response help us to locate where an animal is on the spectrum of wellness, unwellness, and illness. They also help us choose which remedies to use to help her heal and assess whether she can cope with strong stimulation or needs a gentler approach. This understanding is crucial because if we apply a remedy that creates more therapeutic stress than the patient can handle, we may overwhelm her and do more harm than good.

Each mode has a different implication for a pet's resilience and strength. An individual dog or cat's stress response mode may be influenced, for instance, by genetic stress or the stress her mother experienced while she was in the womb. (See pages 72–73.) However, dietary, environmental, and other stress factors can shift the pet into a stronger or weaker mode than she was born with. Your job as your pet's primary caretaker and your vet's job as your coach is to help your dog or cat move to a better response mode and to not push her into a weaker mode. This is why it's important to appreciate how the modes differ from each other.

HOW MUCH WATER IS IN THE WELL?

To understand the four modes of stress response we can use the analogy of a well. Think of the well as the immune system, and the water in the

Holistic Health Care Is a Better Investment

At times, it may seem more expensive to support the living terrain to function at its highest capacity than to purchase mainstream medications in an attempt to keep the body going even as it breaks down. High-quality food and ongoing therapies such as chiropractic care may appear to cost more up front than some pharmaceuticals. It is true that the holistic way puts great emphasis on prevention; investing the time, energy, and money to prevent future problems can be a front-end-loaded endeavor. But its long-term benefits far outweigh the often temporary usefulness of invasive medications and reduce the likelihood of requiring much more expensive surgeries and high-end drugs down the road. A complete program of holistic care for wellness is a true investment in long-term health, and like any sound investment its payoffs are worth it.

well as energy. The earth around and above it is the living terrain. Imagine that the living terrain near the well has burst into flames, indicating that it is under severe stress. To help it return to homeostasis we need to put out the fire, and to do this we must draw upon the water in the well. The amount of water in the well represents the energy available to the dog or cat's immune system to respond to stress. The various amounts of energy available are reflected in the differences among the four modes.

In **Response Mode 1,** the energy available to the immune system is comparable to the water supplied by a full Artesian well that flows all the time without an apparent limit. The pet in Mode 1 will encounter stressors like any other animal, but she has the energy and ability to put out the average fire very easily without need of additional support. She may visibly react to stress that comes her way, but her capacity to handle it is excellent. When challenged by most stressors, the pet in Mode 1 is likely to experience as interference anything we do to try to help her. There is no need to interfere with an immune response that's more than adequate.

Most pets—as is probably true for most people—are in **Response Mode 2** when facing most stressors. They don't have quite as much water in the well as they would have in Mode 1, so it takes longer to put out a fire. Because the well is not full and flowing, the pet is also more susceptible to recurrences of the same problem. But a pet in Mode 2 can still push back with some strength, and just a little help from us will help her complete her response and resolve the issue. If a stressor is powerful, pets in Mode 2 and occasionally those in Mode 1 may need a little assistance. These animals can handle the extra stress from supportive therapies, so we can use stronger intensities and the problem will clear up in no time. However, I would not use disruptive therapies such as antibiotics with these more resilient animals. I've often seen invasive therapies do more harm than good, for example, by creating dysbiotic stress that complicates the animal's situation.

A pet in **Response Mode 3** has a low water level. She keeps using up what water she has, but she never has enough in reserve to put the fire out. As a result, she suffers from chronic or repeated illnesses and does not respond quickly to the help we may give her. She may also be very sensitive and may react to a stressor with a greater degree of severity than the challenger calls for. This dog or cat needs multilevel support to enable her to overcome the stressors that ail her, but with appropriate assistance she will improve and her response mode may improve, as well.

Finally, in **Response Mode 4** the well is almost dry. This pet has very little ability to fight infections and at the best of times only produces a minimal immune response. Even when she does make some progress she has trouble sustaining it and is soon overwhelmed again by illness. In fact, the pet in this mode has such a weak response that we can say she is close to death. We can technically describe death as the complete absence of response to stress. (See Chapter 9.) When providing therapy for an animal in Mode 4 we must be extremely careful because we do not want to create more stress for her under any circumstances.

A dog or cat in Mode 3 or 4 is depleted, so I would not push these pets with therapies that stimulate their immune systems too much, at least until they begin to show greater resilience. To relieve debilitating symptoms to minimize the animal's stress and give her a chance to rally, I might even use carefully selected, quick-acting mainstream drugs. For example, if a dog or cat in Mode 3 or 4 had a bacterial infection, I might use antibiotics. But I would always do this in the company of supportive measures.

In most cases a pet's response mode will be such that she will benefit from supportive measures of appropriate intensity. But even if a pet is in Mode 4 and is clearly going to die, steps can be taken to smooth her final experience. (See Chapter 9.)

THE FOUR MODES AS A GUIDE TO THERAPY

When Wendy's standard poodle Pierre began to seizure, she rushed him to an emergency clinic. There, she was told that he had an inoperable brain tumor and nothing could be done except to control his seizures to make life more bearable for him until he died. Pierre was put on phenobarbital to control his epilepsy as well as prednisone to reduce the symptoms caused by the tumor and the inflammation around it. Wendy accepted the drugs for her dog, but she did not want to accept the mainstream view that nothing more could be done for him without first investigating a different approach. And so it unfolded that Pierre became one of our patients.

When I took the case, I did not adjust Pierre's drug regime. I don't object to using pharmaceuticals as an emergency measure—for example, to control seizures—but I do not see them as the solution to a problem. They are solely palliative: they help manage the pet's condition but do nothing to improve it. Further, as I mentioned earlier in this chapter, because pharmaceuticals impose change upon the living terrain, they may also create additional negative stress for an animal already struggling with poor health. (Also see Iatrogenic

Stress on pages 81–84.) So while I believe pharmaceuticals have a role in cases like these, therapies that support the living terrain offer an ill pet a lot more.

Just because a pet may have been diagnosed with a condition from which she will probably die—such as a brain tumor—does not mean she is ready to die. In spite of her illness she is still a viable being. Too often, mainstream thinking assumes we can either do nothing but wait for a terminally ill pet to die or euthanize her. But as long as her quality of life is reasonable, we should actively help her to be as well as she can for as long as she can.

When Pierre came into my clinic, he was not ready to die. To lessen his need for palliative drugs while helping him maintain an adequately normal life, we gave a gemmotherapy combination that included Juniperis, Ulmus, and Ribes Nigram to drain his body of toxins. I put all of my prednisone cases on Ribes Nigram because, among other things, it counteracts the suppressive effects of prednisone by stimulating the adrenals to produce steroids naturally. We also tried to improve Pierre's nutrition by feeding him unprocessed foods and supplementing him with antioxidants, omega-3s, and probiotics. On this regime the poodle began to do well—his seizures were under control and he was eating heartily and enjoying life.

Pierre did so well that he appeared to be in Response Mode 2. So we went on to our next goal of trying to improve his response to the stress caused by his tumor. Auricular medicine assessment testing helped us clarify which environmental or dietary stressors to mitigate and which remedies would likely help him. Then we devised a more intense plan based on a different homeopathic complex to continue detoxification plus support his nervous system tissues.

But things did not work out as we had hoped. Pierre began to vomit and have diarrhea and he did not look well. After one more day of doing poorly on the new therapy regime, we took him off it. Pierre bounced back to his previous level of wellness. I interpreted his fast recovery to mean that the more intense therapy had pushed him further than his immune system could cope with—his ability to respond was more of Mode 3 than Mode 2 as it had first appeared to be. We stayed with the nutritional support and let him restabilize.

Pierre was fine for the following week but then started seizuring again. Wendy took him to the emergency clinic once more, where his phenobarbital was slightly increased to bring the seizures under control. Then she brought Pierre back to me. This time, we introduced a different set of homeopathic remedies tailored to work more gently with his weaker response mode. It worked. We struck the balance we sought, and Pierre improved enough to enjoy a reasonable quality of life until his time came, more than a year later.

Sometimes it's hard to know whether an apparently negative response is part of a necessary adjustment the animal is making or whether he's simply not strong enough to handle the therapy we're giving him, and Pierre's case was challenging in this regard. Fortunately, he stabilized nicely once we stopped pushing him so hard. This is another benefit of the supportive remedies: because they do not attack the living terrain, they tend not to permanently damage it, even when given to an animal who cannot handle their intensity. In a case like this the trick is to recognize when to back off.

I choose each course of therapy according to which modalities will be most effective for the pet's particular problems and which stress response mode I perceive him to be in. I take into account his appearance, the client's description of his symptoms, and the results of any physical, biochemical, and bioenergetic tests we may carry out. Once we have begun the therapy, I remain available to the client and adjust the type and intensity of the therapies we use according to the pet's subsequent reaction to them. My goal is to help the animal as much as possible without overwhelming him.

When Caleb had distemper, for example, we considered that his response mode had likely been weak to begin with, which was why he had been susceptible to disease. Because we did not want to risk over-whelming him with a remedy that might be too strong for his living ter-rain to handle, we advised Susan to start him on a weaker potency first and watch for signs of improvement. Caleb responded beautifully—the lower potency proved to be enough to save his life. If we'd given him a higher potency or otherwise tried to energize him too heavily, we might have put him into greater difficulty and the therapy would not have been beneficial. I follow this guideline with all my cases.

YOU ARE YOUR PET'S CLOSEST OBSERVER

When recommending a plan of action to help an animal recover, I explain my choices to my clients in terms of how much therapeutic stress I think a pet can take. But again, because you are the person who knows Esmeralda most intimately, your observations, intuition, and input into the decision-making process are crucial. Whenever your pet is under *any* kind of therapy—whether supportive or mainstream—watch for significant signs of change in her energy level, behavior, inter-est in life, and physical signs, such as those listed on pages 128–130 under The Early Signs and Symptoms of Unwellness. If you think she is getting worse, give your vet that feedback right away. When a sup-portive therapy appears to be overwhelming a patient, the client and I work together to back it off a bit, call it off entirely, or change our approach altogether. Although when using supportive therapies an apparent worsening of symptoms may sometimes indicate a healing crisis (see pages 31–32), this judgment call must be made carefully every time. On the other hand when a mainstream therapy seems to be overwhelming the patient, an urgent response may be called for. A patient going into anaphylactic shock after receiving an antibiotic or immunization is a good example: in such a case, an immediate anti-dote or other emergency support would be required to save her life. Trust your observations and get help when you think you need it. If your vet does not seem to be interested in taking your observations and concerns into account, you can and probably should seek out a second opinion.

APPLYING THE FOUR MODES TO EVERYDAY LIFE

Finally, I advise my clients that the four modes of stress response need to be taken into account when deciding which habits of daily living will suit the pet. Taking exercise as an example of a stressor, if a pet is by nature a couch potato, she should be treated as such. A typical cocker spaniel or Irish wolfhound who loves to rest by your side should not be expected to exercise with great vigor as a Border collie might need to do. To do so could push her too far. An active dog who is a born athlete will turn the experience of heavy exercise into a positive stress and will turn inadequate exercise into a negative stress, whereas a more compromised individual will benefit from exercising lightly but will turn heavy exercise into a negative stress. (See pages 102–105 for more on exercise.) Be realistic about your pet's ability to respond, and give her opportunities to interact with stress that is appropriate for *her.*

Some health care problems are more challenging than others. Chapter 8 shows how supportive remedies really shine in some of the toughest cases pets, pet lovers, and veterinarians ever have to face.

ENDNOTES

1. See, for example, Wendell O. Belfield, DVM, and Martin Zucker, *How to Have a Healthier Dog: The Benefits of Vitamins and Minerals for Your Dog's Life Cycles* (San Jose, CA: Orthomolecular Specialties, 1981), 245; and Richard Pitcairn, DVM, and Susan Hubble Pitcairn, *Dr. Pitcairn's New Complete Guide to Natural Health for Dogs and Cats,* 2nd ed. (New York: Rodale Books, 1995), 258.

2. Ascorbic acid can be too harsh for a dog's stomach so Susan used sodium ascorbate, which she happened to have on hand. But sodium ascorbate can be difficult to find. Calcium ascorbate is more readily available and is an ideal choice for dogs.

3. I sometimes use these other terms because the English language hasn't yet caught up with the changing health care landscape. Please take this as my nod to established terminology, but do not let it confuse you about my position.

4. Nambudripad's Allergy Elimination Techniques (NAET®) is a complex and interdisciplinary approach to eliminating sensitivity to allergies that employs acupuncture and acupressure among its techniques.

5. This approach differs from how therapies such as pharmaceuticals are administered, where the correct dosage is usually based on an animal's body weight, the cycle of the substance itself, and the disease the animal is perceived to have.

6. Many homeopaths have adapted the concept of these response modes to fit with their refinement of homeopathic theory. A classic example of someone who has contributed enormously to this body of knowledge is James Tyler Kent. See James Tyler Kent, "The Science and the Art," in *Lectures on Homeopathic Philosophy,* reprint edition (Berkeley, CA: North Atlantic Press, 1979), 121–51.

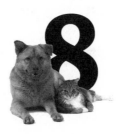

An Approach to Three Health Care Nightmares

Of all the health issues their pets may have to deal with, my clients dread allergies, autoimmune illnesses, and cancer the most. Each of these challenges is a nightmare for the patient, the people who love him, and the vet who wants to help him, and each appears to set into motion a downward spiral from which the pet is unlikely to return. People often believe that allergies only get worse, that autoimmune illnesses will devastate the body, and that cancer is a death knell.

They also worry that treatments for these conditions will be hard on their animals. Mainstream treatments can be painful, may continue indefinitely, and may significantly decrease the patient's quality of life. For instance, allergy shots are sometimes administered for a long time. Complicated autoimmune treatments may require procedures that the animal doesn't like. Surgery to remove cancerous parts of the body can disfigure and compromise an individual's wellness as much as or more than might the malignant growth itself. And chemotherapy can cause pets a great deal of suffering or even death, and often doesn't stop the cancer anyway. Considering all the factors involved, once a pet has been diagnosed with one of these conditions, a client will often fear that there's no hope for her beloved companion but to be taken down by the illness.

But from my perspective we can look at allergies, autoimmune illnesses, and cancer in a much more hopeful and helpful way. By viewing them through a stress-based holistic lens, we can obtain a different understanding of what they are, their underlying causes, and what we can do about them.

To obtain this new understanding, we must become less concerned with the biological origins of these conditions and more open to using whatever approach will work, even if we can't fully explain *why* it works. Although all kinds of theories and billions of research dollars have gone into figuring out exactly what makes people and animals develop allergies, autoimmune illness, and cancer, nobody knows the answer. And they continue to cause a great deal of suffering in spite of the hard-hitting mainstream methods created to relieve them. As a practicing veterinarian who sees animals with these terrible conditions every day, I am more preoccupied with finding a way to address them that is both safe and effective. Over many years, I have developed an approach that has benefited my patients significantly.

My multifaceted plan of action to address allergies, autoimmune illnesses, and cancer is based on the philosophy I laid out in Chapters 1 and 2, which asserts that stress underlies every health care issue and that energy must flow freely to achieve wellness. I also believe that we can manage these health disasters better if we have a way to understand them. So I have developed a practical way of explaining these conditions to clients whose pets are thus afflicted. The explanation that I give to my clients is the one that I offer in this chapter. I do not intend it as a contribution to scientific theory, nor do I present the approach I have created as a magic answer to these problems. There *is* no magic answer. But the approach I have developed has produced remarkable results, including in some cases the conditions disappearing altogether. In other cases, dogs and cats who could not completely recover have suffered less and lived longer than would have typically been the outcome.

Allergic Reactivity

Megan had already tried all kinds of mainstream methods by the time she first brought Moira, her West Highland white terrier, to see me. The four-year-old dog's skin was red and itchy, and she had lost hair from her flanks and around her eyes. She frequently chewed at her feet and pawed at her face.

"She scratches herself all the time," Megan said. "At first it was just in the summer, but now she's itchy all year. It torments her." I could see how much she longed to help her dog feel better.

I learned from Megan that Moira's diet was primarily kibble and that she was given lots of baked treats—all of which were the best quality Megan could find but heavily processed nonetheless. Every month, to prevent possible infestations of fleas and internal parasites, Megan used an insecticide that is absorbed into the living terrain through the skin. Added to this, her previous clinic had given Moira anti-inflammatory drugs and antibiotics many times to treat her skin symptoms. But the problem kept coming back and getting worse.

Moira appeared to be a typical allergically reactive dog. From a holistic point of view, her living terrain for a long time had been under siege when support was what it desperately needed. Given how severely and persistently allergic she was, I also assessed that her stress response mode was weak—she was probably in Mode 3. (See page 174.) For all these reasons, her immune system spiraled further out of whack while producing symptoms that made Moira miserable.

Moira's symptoms also distressed Megan. "I've heard that skin problems only get worse," she told me. "So I don't expect her to get better, although it would sure be nice if she did! But I don't want her to be on medication for the rest of her life. I hope you can recommend something safer or more natural for her."

Megan's assumption that Moira was stuck with allergies for life was understandable, because this tends to be the outcome when allergy cases are not approached from a holistic perspective. But my experience has been different. "There's a lot we can do," I assured her. "First off, we need to think differently about the situation. Don't think in terms of Moira having a skin problem. Think in terms of her having an immune system problem."

A DISTURBED IMMUNE RESPONSE IS THE CAUSE

I explained to Megan that although Moira fitted the picture of an allergic dog, the diagnosis did not end there. I believe that allergic reactivity is a sign of a deeper problem—a disturbed immune system.

A disturbed immune system can express itself in many forms, as we have seen in stories and case studies in previous chapters. But allergies, autoimmune illnesses, and cancer are arguably the most challenging health crises it produces. They are very difficult to overcome and they frequently cause the animal's physical and emotional state, and therefore his quality of life, to deteriorate. Sadly, veterinarians are seeing more of these health nightmares every day. Mainstream medicine categorizes and treats them as separate conditions based on their different symptoms. But I believe that all three stem from the same underlying problem, which is that stress has negatively affected the immune system in ways that prevent it from doing its job properly. (See pages 52–54 for a description of a healthy functioning immune system.)

I'm not saying that stress disrupts the immune system's function in exactly the same way in each of these conditions. Each condition represents a different kind of immune failure. In allergic reactivity, the immune system mistakenly identifies harmless substances as threats and responds to them in a way that causes damage to tissues such as the skin. In autoimmune illness, the immune system ceases to recognize invasive substances until they have begun to interfere with the living terrain. At this point, it severely attacks those areas of the living terrain in which they have become embedded. In cancer, the immune system stops controlling the division of body cells, which leads in turn to malignant growth. So when a cat or dog has allergies, an autoimmune issue, or cancer, we need to ask how stressors have disrupted, weakened, or otherwise compromised the immune system and what we can do to modify, if not reverse, the process.

In Chapter 3, (beginning on page 71),we looked at eight different realms of stress that weaken the living terrain and undermine the immune system's ability to function normally. In complex cases such as allergic reactivity, autoimmune illness, and cancer, I believe that there are multiple culprit stressors and that their effects have accumulated over time. In other words, allergies, autoimmune illness, and cancer are the final manifestation of an ongoing series of disturbances.

But from a holistic perspective, to return the patient to wellness we don't focus on these final manifestations because they are not the real issue. The real issue is the immune system problems that led to them. Our approach to healing must be to support the disturbed immune system, to track back to the sources of stress that caused the disturbance, and to minimize or remove them altogether.

This is easier said than done. Supporting a disturbed immune system, tracking back to stressors, and modifying or removing them requires a close partnership between the vet and the client. But the client does the heavy lifting. To help her be effective, I believe it is important to take time to explain in lay terms how damage to the immune system produces the particular condition that her dog or cat is experiencing. I regard this as the first step in my eight-point plan to support the immune system. This is the way I explained Moira's allergies to Megan.

ALLERGIES—THE IMMUNE SYSTEM IN OVERDRIVE

Because Moira's immune problem manifested itself as allergic reactivity, I explained to Megan that when the immune system functions normally, various elements, such as lymphocytes, circulate through the living terrain to help it maintain its integrity. Some elements, such as mast cells, congregate in certain tissues that act as major components of the immune system, primarily the skin in dogs and cats and the upper respiratory system in people. From their location in these tissues, mast cells are ready to respond to a foreign invader. As described on page 52, foreign substances that stimulate the immune system to respond are called antigens. When the immune system correctly recognizes an antigen such as a virus or bacteria, it mobilizes its forces to attack. As part of the process, tissue-based mast cells release chemicals such as leukotrienes, inflammatory prostaglandins, and histamines, which cause swelling and inflammation. After a healthy immune system has ousted the invader, it stops attacking and the symptoms its attacks have created disappear.[1]

In my view, in allergic reactions the immune system responds inappropriately to harmless substances that have entered the living terrain, such as pollens or foodstuffs, and treats them as invaders that must be attacked. So the mast cells rapidly release their irritating chemicals, which build up in the tissues in greater amounts than would normally come into play. This is what creates the symptoms that are associated with systemic allergic reactions, such as chronically itchy skin or upper respiratory discomfort.

In dogs, these chemicals tend to build up in the skin all over the body and particularly in the feet and around the face, producing red, inflamed skin and itchiness. This is why dogs who have allergies chew their feet and paw their faces. In cats, these chemicals also accumulate in the skin and the face, but cats often have more pronounced upper respiratory symptoms such as wheezing and inflamed sinuses, leading to a drippy nose and weeping eyes. (Although both dogs and cats may have upper respiratory symptoms, these are much more typical in people.) Both species can also have localized reactions called contact allergies; for example, if a pet is allergic to new bedding, he will develop redness and itching where his skin touches the bedding and possibly elsewhere on his body. And so-called hot spots are a secondary allergic reaction to bacteria that normally live harmlessly on the skin.

Moira's immune system likely mistook everyday substances such as pollens or mold to be invaders and went into overdrive, producing the chemicals that caused her skin to itch. So her itching was not caused by pollens or mold but rather by the chemicals her immune system produced because it misinterpreted these substances as a problem. Over time, as her immune system mistook more substances for invaders and produced more inflammation-causing chemicals, her itching became more constant and intense.

To address this challenging problem, the first question the mainstream approach asks is, "What substances is Moira allergic to?" But the question I care about is, "Why did this pet's immune system start reacting inappropriately and excessively to harmless substances?" My answer is: because of stress.

The kind of imbalance that makes an allergic pet's immune system misfire may be caused by any combination of factors from the eight realms of stress. Genetic stress may often play a role by setting up an inherited weakness. Neonatal stress may prevent the puppy or kitten's immune system from forming correctly. Iatrogenic stress from over-immunization or from drugs, including pesticides, may compromise the living terrain more. Finally, emotional and environmental stressors trigger the problem to express itself. In short, if stress interferes with or alters the immune system, it will malfunction. The pet begins to react to harmless substances, and these reactions may get worse over time. In my view, this is why allergies exist, and it provides the clues to what to do about them.

A MULTIFACETED APPROACH THAT WORKS

You may be familiar with the mainstream approach to treating pets who have allergies. It involves either trying to desensitize the immune system by injecting allergens under the skin, or suppressing inflammation with cyclosporine or corticosteroids. Hot spots are usually treated with antibiotics. But from my point of view, the problem is not the allergen—it's the pet's immune response to the allergen. That's what I work on. Experience has shown me that if we can improve a pet's immune response, her hyperreactivity to stressors, including seasonal ones such as pollens, won't likely return as often or as intensely. The holistic philosophy is to heal from the inside, out.

I believe that a misfiring immune system that produces allergic reactions can be improved by a multifaceted program of holistic support. In a typical week, I see four or five allergy cases. I have been using the approach I describe below since the 1990s, and it gets results.

There's no question that allergies are a really tough problem to solve. But although every individual is different, most of my patients get a heck of a lot better than they were. Some pets have seemingly miraculous recoveries, and others don't improve at all because their immune systems are too far gone for us to help them. But most cases fall somewhere in between. I don't offer false hope; because it's so difficult to help an allergic pet's immune system totally recover its balance, most pets will continue to have some allergies, although they will suffer significantly less than before. But we generally see major improvements.

I put all my allergy patients on the following eight-point plan. It is accomplished over six weeks, with an interim appointment three weeks into the program. The sequence that I follow is very important.

1) Understand the problem. The first thing I do is explain to the client how her pet's immune system is producing the problem, as I did with Megan. If you understand what's causing your pet's allergies, you'll be much better able to support her. This is equally true for autoimmune illness and cancer.

2) Eliminate stress. The next step toward rebalancing the immune system is to eliminate as many stress factors as possible from the dog or cat's life. I ask my clients to think about what kinds of emotional, environmental, or iatrogenic stressors the pet may be dealing with and what they might do to reduce or remove them. (Chapter 3 will jog your mind about the possibilities.) Obviously, we can't control common allergens, such as pollens or mold, for example, but we should reduce or remove stressors we *can* control. If we don't reduce the pet's stress, she'll never get better and her problems will manifest in another way.

To help Megan reduce environmental toxins and potential iatrogenic stress for Moira, I recommended that she stop treating her with the monthly systemic insecticide she'd been using. In my view, pesticides should not be utilized except as a short-term emergency measure when a pet has an overwhelming infestation. For example, given the region I live in, I don't recommend heartworm preventive for my patients, and they have not developed heartworm.[2] Megan and I discussed alternative ways to discourage pests, ranging from herbal methods to—as a last resort—occasional use of monthly insecticides that, unlike her previous kind, are not absorbed through the skin.

On the emotional side, Megan told me that because she worked at home, Moira was always with her. But lately Megan's mother was ill, so Megan often had to leave during the day to drive her mother to health care appointments. She couldn't take Moira along because the dog liked to chase her mother's two cats. Megan had noticed that Moira seemed confused and bewildered about her sudden comings and goings. She decided to try structuring at least twenty minutes of focused playtime with Moira every day to see if it might relieve her anxiety. I also gave her a flower essence to help the dog cope with this emotional stressor.

3) Palliate symptoms. Severe or relentless pain or discomfort can burden an animal with additional stress and prevent her from having the rest periods she needs in order to recover. (See pages 47–48.) For example, severe skin irritation and constant scratching can keep a pet from sleeping properly and giving her skin a chance to mend. Whenever possible, I relieve intense symptoms such as these with noninvasive remedies that do not suppress the immune system but gently encourage it to improve. In the worst cases, I will prescribe an anti-inflammatory drug such as prednisone to give the pet a break and allow her to get some rest, but I will limit its use to just a few days.

For Moira, I supplied a homeopathic salve that calms the immune system's inflammatory response.

4) Put the pet on an unprocessed diet. Because good food is the mainstay of support for the living terrain, I switch the patient to an unprocessed diet right away. The diet must be grain-free, and for allergy cases I make sure the client excludes beef as a protein source because many animals have a sensitivity to it. We will take further steps to figure out which foods, if any, the pet is sensitive to, but this is a place to start. I counseled Megan on how to feed Moira this way and supplied her with printed guidelines. (See The Stress-Busters Diet for Dogs and Cats in the Appendix.)

5) Balance gastrointestinal flora. I put all of my allergy, autoimmune, and cancer patients on probiotics to improve their digestive function with helpful bacteria because a well-functioning GI tract has a profound effect on a healthy immune system. These supplements help to balance the GI tract in the short run and support its efforts to rebalance itself in the longer run.

The five points above are fundamental to my plan of action for animals who suffer from allergies, autoimmune illness, or cancer. I have the client implement them right away, and they work very well to start shifting the animal's underlying condition. But this part of the plan works even better once it is refined to meet the needs of the individual. There are two ways to do this. My preferred way is to have the pet bio-energetically assessed. (See The Beauty of Bionenergetic Assessment on page 148.)But if the client cannot or will not agree to this, then we use trial and error to find out which combination of foodstuffs and remedies will best help the pet. Both ways will get us there, but bioenergetic assessment will get us there much quicker.

6) Bioenergetic assessment. Bioenergetic assessment gives us a heads-up about which foodstuffs and remedies trigger an inflammatory response in the pet, and which ones she reacts to positively. This is important because giving a reactive pet a remedy or food to which she is sensitive can do more harm than good, and knowing which ones she will respond to positively is a boon to her recovery. I don't see the point of testing for ubiquitous environmental allergens, such as house-dust mites, ragweed pollen, and so on; we focus on supporting the immune system instead. Bioenergetic assessment also tells us which organs or tissues are blocked up with toxins and would therefore benefit from drainage remedies.

Megan decided to proceed with auricular medicine assessment for Moira, so my next step with her was informed by the results of the testing. It showed that Moira responded well to turkey, duck, and chicken and reacted negatively to beef, lamb, carrots, potatoes, and beets. She appeared to be fine with a variety of other vegetables. I advised Megan to revise Moira's diet by drawing solely from items on the positive list and avoiding those on the negative list. We also explored Moira's responses to various drainage remedies and tonics.

7) Drainage and detoxification. Complex, low-potency remedies help cats and dogs with disturbed immune systems clear out the toxins that create biochemical and energy blockages in their living terrains.

Although I use homeopathy for this purpose, acupuncture can provide an alternative approach if the client prefers it.

Auricular medicine assessment revealed that Moira had toxic buildup in her liver and kidneys and that she responded well to gemmotherapy drainage combinations containing Juniperis and Ulmus, as well as to certain Unda complexes. And although I do not normally utilize herbal remedies with allergy patients lest they become reactive to them, Moira's results showed that she was fine with milk thistle, an herb that is very useful for detoxifying the liver.

8) Tonics. I use nutritional supplements such as vitamins, essential fatty acids, and so on for secondary assistance when an individual appears to require more help than dietary and GI changes plus drainage remedies can provide. Generally speaking, tonics such as these are designed to contribute additional supportive material to the living terrain. They can enhance a holistic plan that is based on an unprocessed diet and a healing system such as homeopathy or traditional Chinese medicine. They can also make up shortfalls for a deficient living terrain that cannot regain its balance in spite of our best holistic efforts. But these tonics cannot help the living terrain become self-sufficient and self-regulating.

Auricular medicine assessment showed us that Moira was highly reactive to both salmon oil and flaxseed oil—a valuable thing to learn about this individual because these oils would otherwise offer excellent support to an allergic dog. On the other hand, although she had a mildly positive response to vitamins E and C, we reasoned that the unprocessed diet might do enough for her on its own. Time would tell whether we should add the vitamins to the plan.

After discussing Moira's test results with Megan, I provided her with a printout along with the drainage remedies and milk thistle preparation. She was eager to see whether our approach would make a difference. I told her that it usually takes time to bring a disturbed

Use Supplements Only When Necessary

Part of establishing an effective plan for healing requires being able to learn continually about what works and what doesn't work for the individual patient. We need to keep therapy simple and straightforward so that we can observe this as we go along. Introducing too many biochemical substances—even supportive ones—into the living terrain can prevent us from seeing whether dietary changes and drainage remedies are doing their job. And because tonics may relieve symptoms in the short run, they can also obscure the need for a more complete approach and delay the patient from starting it. I believe that whenever possible, our goal must be to help the living terrain become more self-sufficient for the long haul, rather than prop it up in the short run.

immune system into better balance and that she should see some general improvement over the next three weeks. She would probably first notice Moira's itchiness decreasing slightly and the dog would appear less agitated.

FOLLOW-UP

Three weeks in. I ask each client who has a pet suffering from allergies to come in for a follow-up three weeks after she has made all of the initial changes. At this time, I check the animal for signs of progress or lack of progress. The client usually has new questions about working with the diet and what else to expect. I reiterate what we're trying to do based on the results of the auricular medicine assessment and explain our goal again because the better a person understands what we're doing, the better she can work with it. We usually don't adjust the plan at this point.

Six weeks in. Six weeks after we begin, we do a second follow-up appointment. The drainage remedies will have done their job by now. On the happy occasions when the pet has entirely recovered, I stop the therapy side of the plan and advise the client to keep up the unprocessed diet and lifestyle changes that underpin the deep shift that has taken place in the animal's immune response. More typically, the cat or dog will be somewhat better but not completely cleared. In these cases, I redo auricular medicine assessment because the pet's reactions will have changed and the new test results will show us where we need to tweak the diet and the therapy.

At the three-week mark, Moira was doing very well and I was confident she would continue to get better. She seemed happier and more relaxed, and although she was still scratching, she no longer did so constantly. The fact that she was still itchy had Megan worried that Moira might not be healing as much as we had hoped; many of my clients share similar concerns at this stage. But the holistic perspective recognizes that healing happens from the inside out. As the pet's immune function improves, the most external organ—the skin—will be the last to recover. I've seen it happen this way time and again, year after year.

THE SAME HEALING PLAN FOR ALL THREE CONDITIONS

I feel great when a pet such as Moira shows overall improvement just a few weeks after we've radically changed her diet and lifestyle. Even if, as in Moira's case, she was still itchy when she came for the three-week appointment, I know from experience that we're making progress and will likely make more. Sometimes, a pet's skin clears up completely, which is very exciting.

What is even more exciting is that not only do my allergy cases respond positively to this multifaceted approach, but so do the patients who have autoimmune illnesses and cancer. It's no puzzle to me that the same approach would work for all three conditions. As I've already explained, allergies, autoimmune illnesses, and cancer are but different expressions of the same underlying problem—an immune system that, for whatever reason, has gone out of whack. So I use the same eight-point

What to Do If You Can't Get Bioenergetic Assessment

My *ideal* plan of action to support an allergic pet—as well as pets with autoimmune illness or cancer—includes bioenergetic testing. But what if, for whatever reasons, bioenergetic testing is not an option for you? There is still much you can do for your pet. Switch to a diet of unprocessed foods and put him on probiotics. Don't give him the foods that pets are most likely to be sensitive to. (See The Stress-Busters Diet for Dogs and Cats in the Appendix for guidelines.) Consider what kinds of stress your pet may be experiencing (use Chapter 3 to get started), and think creatively about what you can do about them. These steps are the cornerstone of animal wellness and they will help most animals who have wonky immune systems improve significantly. Once these measures are in place, if you have access to one, a holistic veterinarian may be able to provide drainage remedies to help your cat or dog rid himself of toxins. And if, in the future, bioenergetic testing becomes available for your pet, you can customize his diet for his individual needs and help him that much more.

healing plan that I used for Moira—adapted to the individual's needs—for every animal that comes into my clinic with one of these nasty conditions, and I consistently get significant results. I will show you next how supporting a damaged immune system in this way has worked for dogs and cats who have suffered from autoimmune illnesses and cancer.

Autoimmune Conditions

Lynda and Yoshi brought in Nero, their black Lab, because the unfortunate fellow had had recurrent diarrhea for months. His diet had always consisted of processed food. His previous vets had attempted in vain to straighten him out by trying him on many processed diet formulations, including special prescription foods made for veterinarians to dispense. Conscientiously covering all possible bases, they had also tried antiparasitical drugs and antibiotics. Still, Nero didn't improve. Neither an endoscopic examination nor a biopsy offered any further clues to the cause of the problem. Nonetheless, Nero had been diagnosed with inflammatory bowel disease (IBD). To their credit, Lynda and Yoshi refused to give up. Even though they had spent thousands of dollars to help Nero to no avail, when someone told them about my clinic, they decided to give us a try.

I explained to them that IBD is not a diagnosis, although mainstream medicine refers to it as a diagnosis. Rather, IBD is a catchall term used to describe a variety of symptoms that appear to have no explanation, including recurring or persistent diarrhea. As well, it is often regarded as an autoimmune condition; whether it truly is or not is the focus of academic debate. In the autoimmune theory of IBD, the immune system would have failed to recognize toxins as they entered the living terrain and they would have made their way to the lining of the gut and embedded themselves there, thus compromising the gut's function. However one explains it, IBD is extremely common. I see it all the time and have found it to be very treatable.

From a stress perspective, the symptoms dubbed IBD indicate a dysbiotic gut—a condition where the flora in the digestive tract are out of balance. (See Dysbiotic Stress on page 74.) A secondary stressor then provokes the dysbiotic gut, which responds by becoming inflamed. I told Lynda and Yoshi that in perhaps 90 percent of my patients, I have found that the secondary stressor that provokes the inflammation is the pet's sensitivity to particular foods. Further complicating Nero's picture were the antibiotics he had been receiving, which I assumed had made his dysbiosis worse.

Although I could use prednisone to control Nero's symptoms, I told them that I didn't want to because steroids slow down the immune system, which has other important jobs to do such as controlling cancers from developing. Instead, I said we needed to start by getting rid of toxins in the living terrain. Our first step would be to put Nero on unprocessed food right away and see whether it made a difference for him.

After a few days of eating solely unprocessed foods, Nero's diarrhea cleared up completely. His response was typical of my patients. I have found that the unprocessed diet improves or clears many cases of IBD without the need to take any other measures. But I do not interpret the resolution of symptoms, no matter how happy an event, to mean that we have solved the underlying problem of the immune system imbalance. And unless we address the underlying problem, the dog or cat will probably tend to manifest the same problems again.

To prevent the pet from becoming sensitive to something new, I believe we should do our best to rebalance the immune response by improving the living terrain. I use complex homeopathic drainage remedies to motivate the body to purge itself of toxins in the same way as I do when an immune disturbance expresses itself as allergic reactivity. When it's available, bioenergetic assessment offers tremendous shortcuts for detecting which foods the pet is sensitive to, and points us to the remedies that his living terrain can benefit from the most. Botanicals can play a role with IBD, too: when digestive symptoms don't resolve as easily as Nero's did, I recommend a blend of herbal gastrointestinal soothants, of which slippery elm will be a key component.

AUTOIMMUNE ILLNESS ATTACKS ITS OWN TERRAIN

Autoimmune conditions are horrible. I feel for those who have them. In this form of immune system disturbance, the immune system fails to recognize an antigen such as a virus or another toxic element. These stressors enter the body, get past the immune system, and lodge themselves in specific cells. There, they interfere with the site's function. Now the living terrain's chemical messengers tell the immune system that it has a big problem, and it strongly reacts. Its response produces chronic inflammation at the site and also attacks the body's own cells, which it should not be doing.[3] To illustrate this, when toxic stressors embed themselves in the gut lining, as in Nero's case, they produce inflammatory bowel disorder; in the joints, they produce rheumatoid arthritis; and in the pancreatic cells, they produce certain types of diabetes.[4] Genetic stress may play a role in creating the weakness in the areas that would admit toxic stressors.

Although I see more dogs than cats with autoimmune illnesses, both species are affected by them. Autoimmune illness manifests in many forms. Although mainstream medicine tends to regard and treat the forms as separate diseases according to the different symptoms they display, I believe that their most important aspect—and the factor we must address to catalyze their healing—is the immune disturbance that lies at their root.

Here are a few examples of autoimmune illnesses that I see in my patients. I follow the same basic healing plan for each form and add specific therapies, such as herbal GI soothants for inflammatory bowel disease, as each situation requires.

Anal fistulas. Mainly found in German shepherds.

Autoimmune hemolytic anemia. Involves fatigue, weakness, can be life threatening. Found in both dogs and cats.

Autoimmune skin conditions. Pemphigus, for example, involves large blisters. Found in both dogs and cats.

Inflammatory bowel disease. Found in both dogs and cats.

Interstitial cystitis. Blood in urine; chronic inflammation of bladder tissue. Found mainly in cats.

Lupus. Found in joints or kidneys; can cause an inflammatory reaction in a variety of tissues. Found in both dogs and cats.

Myasthenia gravis. Affects neuromuscular junctions; causes weakness. Probably more common in dogs.

Rheumatoid arthritis. More common in dogs.

Stomatitis. Ulcers at the back of the mouth degenerate; goes into the bone tissue. Found in cats only.

Type 1 diabetes. Destroys beta cells of pancreas. Found in both dogs and cats.[5]

TIMMY, A CAT WITH INTERSTITIAL CYSTITIS

Timmy had blood in his urine. The gray tabby had already seen five vets and been on as many antibiotics, but his problem had not yet been solved by the time Laurel brought him to me. Standard tests, including X-rays and an ultrasound, showed no tumor or bladder stone that would explain his bloody urine, but they did show that his bladder wall had thickened. This left us to suspect a condition that we refer to as interstitial cystitis. No one really knows what causes it in cats, but it's similar to an autoimmune illness that people get. In cats it typically involves chronic inflammation of the bladder wall.

When I asked Laurel if anything had changed in Timmy's life around the time he developed the problem, she told me that she and her husband had adopted a new dog. The dog was not aggressive, but Tommy sneaked around the house very carefully, indicating to me that his new canine housemate was causing him to be stressed out emotionally. He probably also had dysbiotic stress due to the antibiotics he had taken over the past few months.

We switched Timmy to an unprocessed diet, added probiotics, and started him on drainage homeopathics that targeted his bladder as well as major organs. We gave him nutraceutical supplements, including cranberry extract; glucosamine (bladder cases are often deficient in this); and antioxidants. Laurel created a sanctuary for him in the house and to feed him on a high shelf so he could feel safe from the dog while he ate. I gave her flower remedies to help with his anxiety.

After six weeks of the new diet, therapy, and lifestyle changes, Timmy's cystitis cleared up perfectly. As a bonus, he and the dog had begun to make friends.

REX, A CAT WITH STOMATITIS

Stomatitis is one of the nastiest conditions a cat can get. My patient Rex was a typical case. He'd been an unkempt and underweight stray when Young Mee had taken him in off the street. She noticed right away that he had difficulty eating and did not gain any weight. Young Mee did not wait long before she brought him in.

Poor Rex had all kinds of symptoms. He had advanced gingivitis and tooth decay. His breath was appalling. When I tried to look inside his mouth I could see that it was terribly painful for him to open his jaws. I quickly realized that Rex had stomatitis, a condition in which the mucous membranes at the back of the mouth become severely ulcerated. I feel so bad for cats who have this condition. They really suffer.

Rex also tested positive for feline immunosuppressive virus (FIV). FIV is not an autoimmune illness, but it makes the pet vulnerable to developing them. FIV is a virus that stresses the immune system, causing it to become unbalanced. As it compromises the immune system, an opportunistic organism can invade the living terrain. The stressed immune system then attacks the tissues in which the invader has become embedded, thus producing the mouth ulcers associated with stomatitis.

Although cats who have stomatitis desperately need support for their living terrain, I've found that they also benefit from drastic intervention to help break the foothold unfriendly bacteria have gained. So we surgically remove the patient's degenerating teeth and put him on antibiotics right away. Then we implement our standard plan for healing: we put him on unprocessed foods and use homeopathics both to drain away toxins and to motivate the immune system to push back against the underlying virus. We supplement him with antioxidants and lots of probiotics. I use the antibiotics on and off for a while, because it takes a long time to repair this kind of damage. In my experience, cats with stomatitis respond very well when antibiotics are part of their overall healing plan; without antibiotics, they don't do well at all. We use them for as long as they are needed while maintaining all the supportive therapies and the unprocessed diet.

Very gradually, Rex recovered. Over six months he gained weight and filled out, began to show zest for life, and became playful and affectionate with Young Mee. His mouth cleared up completely, to our great relief. Because we could not be certain whether he had overcome the FIV, he would have to be monitored for the rest of his life—if it still lurked in his system he could once again develop stomatitis or other secondary complications. Luckily, Young Mee was devoted to him. She was prepared to keep him on the unprocessed diet and to remain vigilant for any sign that he might need our help again.

As troublesome as allergies and autoimmune conditions are to both pets and their human companions, cancer is the condition that strikes the greatest fear in the heart of pet people and challenges their ability to have enough hope to stick with a healing plan.

Cancer—The Immune System Loses Control

Cancer is a failure of the immune system to control cell division properly, which results in invasive and destructive growth.[6] In my view, the immune system disturbance that leads to cancer is caused by stress. With cancer, as with allergic reactivity and autoimmune illness, a combination of stressors is the probable cause of why the cells begin to function abnormally, and these include genetic and environmental factors as well as others.

Abnormal cell division can be minor, such as a simple nodule in the skin, and has little significance to the patient's overall health picture as long as the immune system contains it in that format. But it can also occur in a more sensitive location, such as the brain, liver, kidney, or blood, where it affects and can destroy the function of the organ.

A simple nodule in a superficial environment such as the skin can be easily removed, whereas out-of-control cell division in a critical part of the living terrain can be difficult or impossible to remove without causing major additional destruction to the area. A cancerous growth is obviously much more difficult to discover when it's internal. But whether it is a simple nodule contained within the skin or an explosion of cellular growth in an internal organ, we must motivate the immune system to take control again the way it should.

We have two goals with cancer: to get rid of the malignancy and to prevent it from spreading. To get rid of an existing growth, we need to look at why it's there and why the immune system did not respond to it. To stop it from spreading or developing again, we must make the immune system recognize the problem and take control of it.

What cancer is all about is simple, really. But for many reasons, we tend to relate to this devastating condition as though it's some kind of horrific mystical disease, and within that framework we want to find its so-called cure. I think the search for a cure for cancer is barking up the wrong tree. If cancer is a failure of the immune system, then to me the answer is clear: support the immune system and help bring it back to a better balance. To achieve these goals, I follow the same multifaceted approach for my cancer patients that I use for allergies and autoimmune illness.

Most of my cancer patients show significant improvement, and they often live longer and with better quality of life than pets who receive mainstream treatment. In a few cases, the pet is not able to respond enough to make the needed difference. On the other hand, I have had cases where the animal's cancer appears to clear up completely. Once again, I am not giving you a magic answer based on a particular recipe of remedies. Just as it is with allergies and autoimmune illnesses, the answer to cancer is not a specific set of therapies but an overall approach that arises out of a different way of thinking whose aim is to support the living terrain.

TARA, A WHEATEN TERRIER WITH SPLENIC HEMANGIOSARCOMA

Hemangiosarcoma is a very aggressive blood cancer that affects the spleen, pericardium, or heart. Sadly, pets who develop the splenic version often die within six to eight weeks of diagnosis. However, many of our patients who've had this affliction have lived a lot longer than that. Tara, Debbie's soft-coated wheaten terrier, is a typical case.

Tara came to us as an older dog. I could see from her medical records that she'd had major allergies all her life, which indicated that she had had immune issues from early on. She'd received all the standard vaccinations a number of years in a row, including one for Lyme disease, even though it is rare in our region. She'd been troubled by hot spots, had eye and ear inflammations, and had at various times been given antibiotics, anti-inflammatory steroids, and cyclosporine. I suspect that all of these factors contributed to the cancer that she eventually developed.

To support Tara's immune system, Debbie arranged for an auricular medicine assessment and we started the dog on homeopathics and probiotics. However, Tara was anemic. We were also concerned about her spleen, which had been enlarged for some time before she came to me, and which continued to get bigger. After ultrasound confirmation, we did exploratory surgery and found two masses on her spleen, so we removed the spleen. The pathology report came back with a diagnosis of hemangiosarcoma, which appeared not to have metastasized.

Splenic hemangiosarcoma has a very poor prognosis as a rule. When the pet's spleen is removed but nothing else is done, the median survival time is from 19 to 86 days, or roughly from three weeks to three months. When the spleen is removed and the animal is treated with chemotherapy, median survival time is 117 to 179 days or four to six months.[7] Debbie preferred not to use chemotherapy but to follow an immune-supportive plan instead.

The drainage remedies we chose for Tara were targeted to blood disorders and cellular degeneration. We gave her another remedy to protect her veins as well as the sodium ascorbate form of vitamin C. She received CoQ10 to tie up free radicals in her muscles and other tissues. We also gave her a special blend of powdered mushrooms designed to activate the natural killer cells in the immune system, modified citrus pectin to try to stop malignant tumors from spreading, and N-Acetyl-L-Cysteine to help control cancer cell development.

As we pushed Tara's immune system to control potential new cancer cells, her allergy-related hot spots then got worse. About two months after her diagnosis, we did auricular medicine assessment again to see Tara's current picture. This pointed us to a whole new group of homeopathics and tonics, and at last Tara's skin calmed down a bit.

Eight months post-diagnosis the dog was still enjoying her life in spite of her persistent skin problems, and there was no evidence of any new malignant growth.

After this, I didn't hear from Debbie for a couple of months, so I figured that Tara had probably died. Prepared for the sad news, I phoned her to ask how Tara was doing.

But Debbie surprised me. "Oh, she's much better," she said. "She's fine!" I was very glad to be wrong. At the time of this writing, Tara's cancer still has not come back. It has been one year since her diagnosis.

Tara's happy outcome is not an isolated event for my clinic. We've had significant successes with this approach. I believe that there's more to our positive results than merely the remedies we offer. In each case, the patient's outcome is directly proportional to her available energy, or in other words, to her stress response mode. The other great influence on outcome is the nurturing attitude of the pet's person. A devoted attitude on the caregiver's part makes a tremendous difference.

LULU, A CAT WITH CANCER OF THE LIVER

From time to time I have the great joy of seeing cancer cases clear up completely. Lulu was one of these cases.

Why I Use Surgery for Cancer

Surgery can save lives in emergencies. An aggressive cancer that spreads rapidly or interferes with an organ or a system's ability to function is an emergency. Surgical removal of the cancerous cells can buy the pet time to allow slower-acting therapies that support the living terrain to do their work. It takes time to shift a disturbed immune system to recover a healthier balance.

Lulu was well into her teens when we first saw her. The pretty white and gray cat had been a stray who found her way into the heart and home of internationally known chef Dinah Koo. When Dinah brought her to us, Lulu looked downright dilapidated. She had not been eating and had been vomiting. She was dehydrated and we could see in her eyes and mouth that she was jaundiced. Her abdomen was extremely tender to the touch.

Because she was in such rough shape, we immediately put her on IV fluids and then ran standard tests to learn the nature of the problem. X-rays showed that Lulu's liver was significantly enlarged. Ultrasound further revealed it contained multiple tumors and that lymph nodes and the abdominal septum were also involved. After ruling out other conditions, we diagnosed her with metastasized cancer of the liver, of which pets normally die very soon after diagnosis. Lulu was in dire straights.

Lulu's overall condition and advancing cancer indicated that she was probably in Response Mode 4. (See pages 174–175.) This meant that we could not be too ambitious with our healing plan; in her weakened state she might easily die from the stress of intense therapy. So we chose a gentle approach, using complex homeopathics for liver drainage and a special blend of dried mushrooms formulated to support a stressed immune system. We based her unprocessed diet on sardine, salmon, and snapper, with vegetables.

Why I Don't Use Chemotherapy

Chemotherapy drugs attempt to destroy cancer cells. They rarely cure cancer but more often achieve a temporary remission that allows the pet's life to be extended for a short period of time. Although these drugs are intended to inflict greater damage to cancer cells than to normal cells, they also damage normal cells. The side effects that follow from this can cause a pet to suffer.

I question the use of chemotherapy because of the damage it inflicts on the pet's living terrain and also because it is very expensive for the client. I prefer the results I see using noninvasive methods that support the living terrain and motivate the immune response to challenge cancerous cells as it should. If a client insists on having her pet treated with chemo, that's her choice, but I won't do it in my clinic. If she finds another clinic that will do it for her, I will continue to support the pet with noninvasive therapy.

All a veterinarian as coach can do is start the client in the right direction and the rest is up to her. Dinah was the one who did the work that kept her cat well. She became deeply involved with learning about, preparing, and experimenting with Lulu's new diet. And from the moment Dinah implemented the healing plan, Lulu got better every day. Six months after her diagnosis we could no longer feel any masses in her abdomen. When pets recover from conditions other than cancer we keep them on the diet but normally stop giving them the supportive remedies. However, when we are making headway with an aggressive cancer, we often recommend that the pet stay on the supportive therapies permanently. In Lulu's case, this meant keeping her on the immune-supportive mushroom blend. As of the writing of this book—a couple of years after her diagnosis—she continues to do very well and the cancer has not reappeared.

It is so rewarding for me, as a holistic veterinarian, to see dogs and cats who have conditions that appear to carry a death sentence return to a greater state of wellness, enjoying the quality of life that their people want them to have. But inevitably, even the healthiest pets reach the point where it is time for them to let go of life, and for us to allow them—or, in some cases, help them—to let go. The next chapter takes a holistic approach to this emotionally painful but nonetheless necessary responsibility that pet lovers must be ready to face.

ENDNOTES

1. Mark H. Beers, ed., "Allergic Reactions," in *Merck Manual of Medical Information, Pocket Books,* 17th ed., 2nd home ed. (New York: Pocket Books, 2004), 1063–73.

2. My region does not have a high incidence of heartworm infestation. This may differ in other regions. However, mainstream thinking is that every pet should receive a monthly preventive, even in regions of low incidence. I don't agree with this stance.

3. Mark H. Beers, ed., "Autoimmune Disorders," in *Merck Manual of Medical Information, Pocket Books,* 17th ed., 2nd home ed. (New York: Pocket Books, 2004), 1073–75.

4. Not all types of diabetes are autoimmune illnesses.

5. Only type 1 diabetes is an autoimmune condition. Dogs mainly develop type 1. Some cats do as well, but cats also have another common version of diabetes that is not a true type 1.

6. Mark H. Beers, ed., "An Overview of Cancer," in *Merck Manual of Medical Information, Pocket Books,* 17th ed., 2nd home ed. (New York: Pocket Books, 2004), 1034.

7. Statistics are taken from Stephen J. Withrow and David M. Vail, *Withrow and MacEwen's Small Animal Clinical Oncology,* 4th rev. ed. (St. Louis: Elsevier Health Sciences, 2007), 791.

PART FIVE

Final
Passage

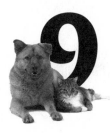

9

Understanding Your Pet's Last Transition

When Maria and Catherine first adopted three-year-old Liberty, they thought she wouldn't live too long. As told in Chapter 1, before she came to them, the rescued Rottweiler had been severely mistreated and had sustained serious injuries when she had been thrown out of a moving van onto a busy highway. But Liberty surprised them and went on to enjoy a long life that was as fulfilling and satisfying as it had been cruel before. I believe that this was due to their love and commitment and to the holistic support that they gave her.

In her new home she joined two dachshunds—Scully and Roonie—and a male Rottweiler called Otto. Liberty soon became the beloved princess of her new household. She also loved to visit the family's farm, where she would sleep and roll in the grass. Luca, a male Rottweiler who joined the family later, became her best friend and she also became close to a female called Kayla. "She enjoyed being the one who called the shots," laughs Maria.

Liberty seemed to bring out caring and kindness in everyone she met. "It was astonishing," said Maria. "She never once growled, bit, snapped, or was aggressive toward anyone, including young children."

The twin boys Aedan and Conor learned to walk by pulling themselves up on her. "She was the sweetest animal you'd ever want to meet."

Liberty's generosity toward and patience with others was remarkable given that her old injuries limited her mobility and must often have caused her some pain. Maria believes that chiropractic care and the other supportive therapies my clinic offered both prolonged the dog's life and gave her greater movement so that she could participate more fully in the family's activities. The other dogs recognized that she could not play as vigorously as they did and found ways to include her in their games. For instance, Liberty would lie with a ball in her mouth and the others would take it, play with it, and bring it back to her. The boys, Aedan and Conor, would roll it to her. That's how the kids learned to roll a ball.

When Liberty was thirteen, Maria called me to say that the dog was in a lot of pain and could hardly get around anymore. Her arthritis had worsened beyond the point where chiropractic adjustments and supportive remedies could help her. She was losing control of her bowels, a circumstance that Maria believed was emotionally difficult for the proud old matriarch to accept. Perhaps most important of all, Liberty had become quiet and no longer seemed to be interested in what was going on around her. "We can see that she's just not there anymore," Maria said. Knowing the dog as she did, she felt that her quality of life had now deteriorated to the point where it would probably be a blessing to end it. I told her to bring Liberty in.

As soon as I set eyes on the old gal I could see that everything Maria had told me was true. The dog appeared to have stopped actively engaging with life. I acknowledged this by saying, "She's very flat." Maria decided then and there to let her go.

Liberty did not resist as I injected the anesthetic. Halfway through the dosage, she quietly departed.

Maria does not regret her decision. "She named the time. We knew she was ready to go. We could have ignored her signals, but Catherine and I just knew."

As the dog passed on, Maria held her in her arms. "I felt that was a gift I had to give to Liberty because she'd given us so much and there was no way I would let her go without me being there to hold her and let her know it was okay. It was hard for me, but it was important."

"She brought a lot of love to a lot of people and did a lot for animal rescue," Maria adds reflectively. "She was a great soul."

We are lucky when, as in Liberty's case, euthanasia is clearly the kind and appropriate thing to do. But in many cases, the appropriate thing to do is not clear. And in some circumstances, I believe that euthanasia is chosen when it should not be.

You will probably agree with me about the kinds of circumstances when euthanasia should not be chosen. We all know of sad, outrageous, and angering cases where people had pets euthanized because the animals were inconvenient to their lifestyles or because they didn't want to take care of them, even though they had the financial means to do so. When a dog or cat is put down for these kinds of reasons, I think it is animal abuse and I have no compunction about saying so. There are so many other options to pursue, including, if necessary, seeking the assistance of one of the many animal rescue organizations that will find another home for a pet who, for whatever reason, no longer fits into its human family's situation. There are many other options, too, for pets who have been seriously incapacitated, as was the case with Brady, the Welsh corgi-terrier cross.

Sometimes There Are Other Options

Brady had an inoperable tumor on his spinal cord, and as a result, he had lost the use of his hind legs. He still had the full use of the front half of his body. In spite of his incapacity, Brady's outlook on life hadn't changed. He was outgoing, interactive, playful, and interested in giving the family cat the evil eye. Most important, he was not in any pain.

Anne and Sabah had taken to carrying him around in a sling. They had considered having Brady euthanized, but it didn't make sense to them to end the life of a dog who didn't seem to be as bothered about his condition as they thought he might be. After all, they reasoned, if Brady was a human being who'd become paralyzed from the waist down, they would not have considered ending his life. Instead, they would put him in a wheelchair and they'd all get on with their lives. So they looked into buying a special cart made to support a dog's back end. With this kind of contraption, Brady would be able to pull himself around using his front legs, and he would regain a fair measure of autonomy and independence. They bought him the cart and were amazed at how quickly he learned to get around with it. The loss of the use of his hind legs was clearly not a problem that Brady found insurmountable once he had a little help from his human friends.

But there are other situations when a dog or cat is affected by a serious condition or injury and people have to confront the question of whether or not to euthanize. The hardest of these situations is when the pet's primary caregiver is faced with a confusing picture.

One common reason for the confusion is that the primary caregiver does not know how the natural dying process unfolds. After all, in Western societies the natural process is often interfered with and is usually hidden out of our sight in hospitals, where our dying loved ones are attended to by strangers instead of by those who are most intimate with them. After death, the body is again attended by strangers. As a result, Westerners typically have little experience with natural death. So, when a pet is dying, the person who loves him tends to believe that he should intervene to save his pet from further suffering, rather than allowing the process to go its natural course. Our lack of emotional experience in dealing with the natural process may also make euthanasia seem to be the choice we would be more comfortable with. For example, Susan started out believing she should interfere when her cat, Abbott, was dying of kidney failure.

The Natural Process of Dying

As told in Chapter 1, at the time he was diagnosed with chronic interstitial nephritis, Abbott, the mottled brown tabby cat, had already begun his decline. When Susan was told that he was going to die, she could have had him euthanized right on the spot. But she decided instead to wait until he truly seemed to be ready to go, and then have it done. So she brought him home to live out his final days where things were most familiar to him and he felt most loved and secure.

After they got home Abbott hid under Susan's bed for a few days, and when he came out again he began to show normal signs of going through the process of dying. First, he no longer seemed to care about whether he ate anything. Susan was able to coax him to take a little food once in awhile, but he finally stopped eating altogether. He began to rest a lot. He still wandered about the house but less often than he used to. On nice days, Susan and Abbott went outside together and she sat with him while he rested in the sun on the back deck.

Earlier in his life Abbott had lived with other people, and from that time he had made another human friend, James, who loved him dearly. Susan thought that James would want to see Abbott one more time before he died, and that it would give Abbott a satisfying emotional experience to spend a few hours with someone he loved in turn and had not seen for a long time. So she invited James over. Although by this time Abbott seemed to only half-care about the everyday events taking place around him, he was glad to see his old friend and spent an hour relating to him before retreating again to lie down by himself. Susan was glad she had arranged this meeting.

Abbott was already very thin, and over the next few days he weakened considerably and became very wobbly on his legs. He slept most of the time, but occasionally wandered around the house, whereas in the past, he had gone outside nearly every day to visit humans and cats who lived nearby. He had a cat friend, a fluffy white male called

Harvey, who used to come around and meow at the kitchen window for Abbott to go outside and join him. But now Abbott stopped going outside the house altogether.

A couple of days before he died he became more lively than he had been for awhile. He wobbled over to the front door to be let out. Susan decided that she would let him go where he wanted to and she would follow him. The tabby slowly and carefully worked his way down the verandah steps and teetered along the short walkway to the sidewalk, where he turned and headed up the street. As weak as he was, he had an air of purpose about him, as though he knew exactly where he was going. Susan walked a few human paces behind him so she could watch over him but not interfere with him.

Two houses away from home, Abbott turned up a driveway and determinedly made his way to a neighbor's back yard where his old friend Harvey often hung out. The two cats greeted each other. Harvey sniffed Abbott over carefully and looked at him for awhile. The woman who lived in the house came out; she was friendly with both cats and she patted Abbott gently. After a little while, Abbott turned around and wobbled back to his own house, where he returned to his place on Susan's bed. It was the last time he ever went out.

The next day, he declined dramatically. He lay on his side, barely moving. Sometimes he seemed to not be present, although he was still breathing. Susan lay beside him, stroking him softly. She wanted him to know that she loved him, but she did not want him to feel as though she was trying to call him back or hold onto his spirit to keep him from going. She kept wondering if now was the time to have Abbott euthanized, but delayed making the call because he did not seem to be in pain anymore and she didn't want to rush him before his time.

At one point Abbott roused himself and tried to get off the bed, so she lifted him down. He lay on his side on the hardwood floor and again seemed not to be present, while Susan rested beside him. Soon after this he let go of the contents of his bladder and a puddle of clear urine grew around him. Susan wiped it away for the sake of his comfort and dignity and gently lifted him onto a towel.

Eventually, she became uncomfortable on the floor but wanted to stay beside him. Hoping that he was past caring where he was, she placed him up on the bed again. Abbott stretched out. After a few minutes, he made a sound from his throat. It wasn't a purr but what we might think of as labored breathing. Then he began to pause between breaths. Finally, he did not take another breath and he was gone. Susan sensed that there was no more life in his body.

The next day, she and a couple of other people who loved Abbott took him to a favorite spot in a ravine and buried him.

The natural process of dying is quite straightforward. As animals near the end of their lives, the energy that flows through their living terrain gradually begins to lessen. They typically show signs of this depletion of energy in the following order. First, they stop grooming or otherwise taking care of themselves. It takes a lot of energy to move the bowels, so they may begin to have problems with house soiling. They stop eating because it takes a lot of energy to digest food, and, rather than living fully, their bodies spend their remaining energy on maintaining a semblance of life.

It's perfectly normal for a dying animal to go for weeks without an appetite. Then, they don't need water anymore, so they stop drinking. Eventually, energy fades from the nervous system, and as this happens they may look dazed. These are normal and natural occurrences.

After a while, negative stress means nothing to a dying pet. Because the body doesn't want to respond to stress anymore, physical discomfort may become a nonissue, and the pet comes to live with it quite peacefully. I've seen this many times; even though a pet may have been in some distress due to illness or a natural degenerative processes, the distress lessens as they move toward death. Near the end, the process actually relieves them of negative stress and they may even appear to enjoy a few days of bliss. At this point it's understandable to think that the pet is having a miraculous recovery, but this is not the case. Rather, the dog or cat is experiencing the final expression of life.

Finally, the living terrain shuts down, the energy flow is depleted entirely, and the body dies. There is no more response to stress. In my view, natural dying, when not accompanied by extreme pain and suffering, does not lead to a bad death. I therefore seriously wonder whether we have the right to intervene in this natural process and bring an end to it prematurely by euthanizing the pet.

Another reason a person may become confused about how to understand and respond to what she sees happening to her pet's body is that other people, such as family members, neighbors, or friends, or information she reads on the Internet, pressure her into thinking that she should euthanize. I've seen many situations where what is happening in the pet's body may look scary and grotesque to the human who loves him but the animal himself is not suffering to the extent that justifies ending his life. Munchkin's story is a good example.

JUANITA'S DILEMMA

Juanita came in with a cat who had a form of cancer that had eaten away the cat's eye and left an empty socket that oozed with discharge. Aside from this alarming feature of his appearance, Munchkin looked bright and interested in where he was and what was going on around him. When I asked her how Munchkin behaved at home, Juanita said he seemed happy and still ran around, playing with his toys and pulling off his usual antics. She said she had brought Munchkin to see me because her friends said she wasn't being fair not to have the cat euthanized in his present condition. Juanita didn't want to have him euthanized, but the pressure she was under made her feel selfish and cruel. She didn't know what to do.

Based on what I could see of Munchkin's condition and what Juanita told me about his attitude toward life, I advised her that Munchkin was not in the kind of pain from which he needed to be rescued with such a

How to Ease a Pet's Natural Death

I advise clients who have chosen to allow their pets to die a natural death to give them the homeopathic remedy Arsenicum Album in the appropriate potency. This remedy is used with people to help alleviate the negative effects of the natural process and help the patient feel better about dying. I can't say that it works for pets as well as it works for people; I have no idea whether it does because the animal can't tell me. But in my experience, most homeopathics do have beneficial effects for animals and at the very least can't do them any harm. Although in various potencies Arsenicum Album may be used for many other conditions as well, to ease the passage into death I use the potency designated as MK.[1]

drastic and permanent measure as euthanasia. "He's still living a normal life," I said, "and he may not ever reach a point of suffering that would call for euthanasia. Why should we take his life before he is ready to go, or at least before the point when it becomes obvious that it would be a kindness to make such an intervention? You are the one who looks after him and knows him best. *You* make the choice for him."

Juanita looked relieved, but she still wasn't sure. "Everybody keeps telling me I should do it," she said. "His eye is gone and he can't see too well out of the other one."

I replied, "It doesn't seem to be bothering *him* that he can't see anymore. He is leading a good life. It's true that he has a gaping wound that looks absolutely gross. It's hard for people to look at!"

Juanita nodded and smiled a little.

"And it's discharging. That's hard to look at too, but in holistic terms discharge is a sign that the living terrain still has some life in it and wants to take care of itself. It's understandable that when a person or an animal looks bad people can wonder how the body could be happy with that mess. But it's his body, and he seems to be fine with it."

Juanita decided not to have Munchkin euthanized but to take him home and let him enjoy himself until his quality of life became significantly impaired, at which point she would think again about whether it would be better to have him euthanized or allow him to die a natural death.

Today, it's almost taken for granted that we should euthanize every pet who is old, ill, or dying. For this reason, people often see or hear that someone else's pet is old or ill and they leap to a conclusion, possibly even taking a moral stance that the pet should be put to sleep. They may take this position without knowing firsthand details about the situation. Most important, they don't live with the animal twenty-four hours a day or know her intimately as the pet's own person does. Unfortunately, it's all too common for people to form strong opinions about things they see or hear of but know little else about, and most of us are probably guilty of doing so at times. But people who have pets—especially those whose pets are old or ill—are often intimidated by this kind of pressure. They may fear that, if they don't euthanize when people tell them they should, they may be guilty of being cruel or insensitive, or of selfishly hanging on too long to their beloved animal friend.

I want to support those of you who have pets to resist this kind of pressure, because I don't believe that we *should* euthanize every pet who is showing signs of approaching the end. Instead, I want to encourage you to make decisions on the basis of your own observations, sound information from your veterinarian, and, above all, your inner sense of what the animal you love needs.

In circumstances like the ones I've described above, euthanasia may not be the most appropriate choice for a pet. But it is clearly warranted when the pet is seriously suffering, as Liberty was, or when the caregiver's own situation has made it impossible for her to provide the care her ill pet needs. In those cases, euthanasia may be the best thing to do.

The Stress of Heroic Measures

When a pet is dying, we need to ask how much stress we will put him through by giving him therapies—whether supportive or mainstream—to keep him going. And when we are able to keep pets alive with artificial means, are we equally able to maintain their quality of life? Because I see dying as a natural process that does not always involve great suffering, I wonder why we choose to keep alive, by artificial means, pets who would otherwise naturally die.

Many of the ways we interfere with pets who are dying are very stressful to them. For example, at a certain point when a pet is naturally dying, he is sometimes put on an IV to maintain his fluid levels as he goes through the process. But this approach no longer makes sense to me. The animal is not in pain; he's simply dying! His energy is depleting, which is a normal part of the process. And as it depletes, he no longer needs to maintain his own fluid levels. So why do we interfere with the process? Further, to carry out this kind of procedure the pet usually needs to be moved from the home into the hospital. But how can a pet who has spent his life in a loving home near his own people possibly benefit from being placed in a strange or frightening environment, in an impersonal clinic, away from the people and perhaps the other animals whom he loves and who love him? What benefits do we gain from doing this to pets? In my view, sending a pet to a veterinary clinic to die is not an appropriate thing to do. The dying pet is better off in the safety and security of his own home.

When you, as a pet's caregiver, reach the point of choosing euthanasia, you will still have decisions to make. Perhaps the most challenging of them is whether you should be present with your pet when he is put to sleep. Yes, whenever possible, you should be with your animal friend, as Maria was with Liberty. It may not be easy, as it was not for Maria. But if your dog or cat is aware of what's going on around him, why would you abandon him now, at the end of a long and happy life together?

Sometimes the pet is beyond knowing whether anyone is present. But even then, for your own sake and just in case he does know, you should be there. And you should always be there if you want to be. In other words, you should not be prevented from being present, nor should you give in to someone else's opinion that you should not be there. This is your decision to make. If you have young children, it is probably best to let them say good-bye to their friend and then have someone accompany them out of the room before your veterinarian begins the euthanization sequence.

There is no right answer to the question of when to euthanize a seriously ill or damaged animal. Different people face different issues of their own. Some may not be able to afford the care that their pet requires. What if the incapacitated dog weighs two hundred pounds and needs to be regularly lifted? Circumstances like these may be the deciding factor, and no one should judge the caregiver when difficult situations that can't be otherwise resolved lead them to euthanize.

My final message to you is a fitting way to end this chapter and this book. In all things, from the minute they enter into your life until they leave it, approach your pets' health care with grace and ease. In a sense, grace and ease is what this book has been about, because it is my attempt to coach you on how to remove whatever stressors may come to interfere with your dog or cat's well-being and enjoyment of life. Sometimes the challenges of unwellness and illness may *seem* complex or difficult, if not insurmountable. But this is not due to the nature of the living terrain and its dynamic relationship to stress. It is due to the approach we bring to it.

The way forward is both simple and practical. The simple speaks to doing things one step at a time for your dog or cat and not doing more than each situation calls for. The practical speaks to not needing to know all the answers to a health problem to be able to do something effective about it.

What I have not done in this book is given you therapeutic recipes or formulas to match up with specific problems. Rather, I've tried to communicate a new way of thinking so that you, in collaboration with your veterinarian, can develop a plan to support *your* pet's wellness, and so you can better understand his unwellness and illness as they arise. *You* are your pet's best friend and caregiver, the number one supporter of his happiness and well-being.

In Conclusion

Your pet is unique. You need each other. Love your pet. Your pet will both receive your love and willingly, selflessly return it many times over. Love is the best stress management tool of all.

ENDNOTES

1. William Boericke, MD, "Arsenicum Album," in *Pocket Manual of Homeopathic Materia Medica*, 9th ed. (Philadelphia: Boericke and Runyon, 1927), 79. Direct quotation: "Gives quiet and ease to the last moments of life when given in high potency."

Appendix

The Stress-Busters Diet for Dogs and Cats

Below are my general guidelines for feeding dogs and cats a balanced, unprocessed diet, as discussed in Chapter 4. For years, my clinic has recommended this simple and straightforward protocol to the great benefit of our patients. Other advocates may tweak the diet a little differently in terms of proportions or contents, and I do not want to suggest that my version is the only way. However, I have found that this uncomplicated, grain-free approach really works. It is an excellent place to begin if you do not have access to a holistic veterinarian who can customize for your pet a diet adjusted to the animal's individual requirements. (See Chapter 6.) If you can consult with a holistic vet who can do this for you, I urge you to do so. The most beneficial diet of all is the one that's tailored to the individual's needs.

For more information or to view my clinic's seminar on homemade diets for pets, visit www.newholisticway.com.

Meat

Both dogs and cats are carnivores. Cats are obligate carnivores, which means they must have meat to survive. Dogs can do well on a wider range of proteins, but in most cases they, too, thrive on a meat-based diet.

Carbohydrates

Dogs and cats do very nicely on protein and fat. They don't require carbohydrates like people do. That said, dogs can handle carbohydrates up to a point, but cats can't deal with them at all well and may develop serious problems on grain-based diets.

THE STRESS-BUSTERS MENU

Every day, dogs and cats need to consume a balanced diet of proteins, vegetables, and fine-ground raw bones. Here's the general breakdown of sources and proportions of each.

Protein sources. Serve chicken, turkey, lamb, rabbit, or fish, and avoid beef.

For animals without known health problems, use this protein-to-vegetable ratio:

Dogs: 50% protein; 50% vegetables

Cats: 75% protein; 25% vegetables

Organ meats. Twice a week, add approximately 10 percent more to the mix in the form of organ meat, such as chicken heart, kidney, or green tripe. You may substitute liver twice a month.

Calcium, magnesium, and other important nutrients. Ground raw bone is an excellent source. Ask local butchers if they'll grind soft, meaty chicken or turkey bones for you, then add some to the veggies and mix. This mix of raw meat, ground bone, and veggies are increasingly available in a prepackaged form, so ask your vet or local pet store if they know of suppliers in your area. If you can't get ground raw bone through either of these means, supply calcium and magnesium either with multimineral tablets suitable for pets or with vegetable greens that are available fresh, in green powders, and in liquid chlorophyll. I recommend avoiding purchased bonemeal because it is difficult to be assured of its purity and quality.

Vegetables. Offer whatever your pet enjoys. Good choices include parsley, broccoli, kale, spinach, romaine, dandelion, and other leafy greens, plus colorful veggies such as carrots, squash, beets, and so on. (See also Foods to Avoid on page 231.) For each meal, mix greens with other colored vegetables to produce combinations such as sweet potato, green beans, and spinach, or broccoli, carrot, and kale. Vary the mix; favor what's fresh and in season. Because dogs and cats' teeth are not shaped for masticating vegetables, these foods need to be gently processed so they can digest them. To prepare veggies, steam them lightly until they're soft or else grate, mash, or blend them to mush, and serve as soon as they've cooled.

A note on grains. Some raw food diets for pets include a substantial portion of grains, but I believe that dogs don't generally need grains, and cats shouldn't have them at all. However, underweight canids may benefit from a weekly supplement of high-glycemic processed grains such as boiled white rice or pasta. Ask your holistic vet to advise you about amounts for your individual dog.

HOW MUCH TO FEED

Providing guidelines for how much to feed pets is challenging because every individual has a different metabolism. The optimal amount for each dog or cat will vary depending on the animal's size, weight, and activity level. What's more, because his activity level will change as his life circumstances evolve, the amount of food he requires will change as well. If you're switching for the first time from commercial food to fresh, unprocessed food, you may also find that your pet needs less food to meet his needs than he required on a processed diet. These amounts are intended as a starting point, after which you may need to make further adjustments according to the instructions below.

Starting point for dogs. Lead off by feeding dogs 2 percent of their body weight in unprocessed food per day. Another way to calculate this is to provide ½ pound (slightly less than 0.25 kilogram) of food per every 25 pounds (11.5 kilograms) of body weight. For example, an 80-pound (36-kilogram) dog would eat approximately 1½ pounds (just under 0.7 kilograms) of unprocessed food each day. Divide the amount into one meal or two, as you and your dog prefer. Dogs can do very well eating once a day, but I've found that most prefer to eat twice.

Starting point for cats. Begin cats on ¼ pound (0.12 kilogram) of food for each 12 pounds (5.4 kilograms) of body weight. Feed cats at least two or three times a day.

Puppies and kittens. In terms of quantity, the guidelines for adult dogs and cats are inappropriate for youngsters. Young animals need an amount of food at least several times greater in proportion to their body weight than the quantity they will need as adults.

Keep in mind that raw foods cannot be left out of the refrigerator for any length of time. If your pet doesn't eat his whole meal at once, you will want to bring out fresh portions for each feeding time rather than leaving out the entire day's ration for her to nibble as she likes.

Adjust amounts according to your pet's hunger level and weight changes. Use your common sense. If your adult pet begins to gain weight, he's getting more food than he needs for his circumstances at this time. Cut back the amount incrementally, observe for a few more days, and adjust again as necessary. On the other hand, if he begins to lose weight or still seems genuinely hungry after meals, he's not getting enough food. In this case, increase the quantity you give him and observe him again to see if it's enough. If not, add a little more and try again. Adjust the amount until you can see that your pet's weight has stabilized and his hunger is satisfied. The amount of food he needs will continue to change as his life changes, so check in with him frequently to make sure he's still getting what he needs. Sharpening your powers

A Healthy Grain of Salt

Don't be taken in by claims that you read or hear about pet foods, pet products, or medical techniques—whether holistic or not—that promise to do wonders for your cat or dog's health.

- Be skeptical of advertising. Its purpose is to make money for business by trying to convince people that a product is perfectly designed to meet their needs.
- Be skeptical of information on the Internet. The Internet proliferates unmonitored, unregulated material, some of which is purely promotional, and some of which is just plain wrong.
- Be skeptical of research statistics. When presented to an unsuspecting audience without proper context or critical discussion, they can be manipulated and portrayed to suggest that almost anything is true.
- Be skeptical of claims of major breakthroughs regarding both natural and mainstream medications and treatments. Only time and experience will tell whether they have any legitimacy.
- Be skeptical of your neighbor's advice. Whether he is a lay person or a professional, he, too, is exposed to information and conditions that may serve an ulterior agenda or motive.

of observation in this way will help you both adjust the amount of food you provide and tune into your pet's health and happiness in general.

RECREATIONAL CHEWING

I recommend allowing pets to gnaw on raw hunks of bone. This does not replace the need for both dogs and cats to consume *ground* raw bone to meet nutritional needs (see above); gnawing on hunks of bone serves a different purpose. It can be very effective in removing plaque from a dog's teeth. It also gives her pleasure, gives her something to do, and provides her with a positive way of discharging emotional stress or tension. Pets may even get some nutritional value from it. *Never* give cooked bones, because they can splinter and become very dangerous inside your pet. Old bones can break teeth and marrow can disturb digestion, so try to find young animal bones, such as veal or lamb. Always supervise dogs while they chew on bones.

Some dogs also enjoy crunching up and eating whole raw carrots, which, like gnawing on recreational bones, can assist in keeping their teeth clean. Although they do not digest raw carrots well enough to draw from them much nutritional benefit, the bits they swallow provide roughage as they go through the intestinal tract.

Heating and Handling

Temperature. You may carefully warm raw food, or gently cook it if your pet insists. I don't believe there's any advantage to cooking it, because both dogs and cats handle raw *meats* very well. However, neither species easily digests raw vegetables, so you'll need to grind these finely. Do not microwave your pet's food! Slow cookers are a convenient substitute for microwaves and preserve nutrients better than almost any other cooking method. Touch food—with your hand, not your mouth—to determine whether it is no warmer than lukewarm. Make certain any chunks or lumps of food are no longer hot *inside*. Be careful not to feed animals from dishes or pans that may still be hot from being used to warm food.

Handle raw meats safely. Take great care preparing and handling raw meats, especially if your own immune system is compromised. Clean surfaces and equipment thoroughly and wash your hands well.

TREATS

To avoid potential problems, keep treats as simple and pure as possible. They should make up less than 10 percent of the pet's daily food ration. I favor plain, dried, unprocessed meats and fish such as chicken, turkey, bison, and salmon. Complicated concoctions that contain many ingredients run a greater risk of courting food sensitivities in your pet and make it hard to detect which stressor the animal has become sensitive to. Keep snacks grain-free; too often I learn that my patients who have obesity problems have been consuming a lot of high-carbohydrate, grain-based snacks every day. Choose unprocessed or only lightly processed treats, such as dried treats that do not contain additives, to reduce the risk of industrial contamination. To control amounts, if you like to give treats often or give food rewards while teaching your dog, then offer smaller pieces each time. Be sure to take into account the amount of treats you give when calculating the total amount of food you provide for your pet each day, and subtract this amount from the main meal.

FOODS TO AVOID

Chocolate, onion, garlic, fava beans, macadamia nuts, grapes or raisins, eggplant, white potatoes, tomatoes, beef, wheat, and corn should not be given to pets. Some of these foods are toxic—even deadly—for dogs or cats or both; others may harm individual animals who may be sensitive to them.

ADDITIONAL SUPPLEMENTS

Essentially, I believe that healthy dogs and cats on an unprocessed diet should not need nutritional supplements. However, for a variety of reasons, even the best foods may not provide enough of certain nutrients. Therefore, I advise adding these to the menu.

For dogs. *Omega-3 oils.* The best sources for dogs are salmon and flaxseed oil. Give smaller dogs a 1,000 milligram gel cap daily; give larger dogs 2,000 milligrams. You don't have to be too precise with amounts of this nutrient; use your best judgement depending on the size and weight of your dog. Prick the gel caps and squeeze the contents onto their food if they will not take them whole.

For cats. *Omega-3 oils.* The best source for cats is fish oil. Give a cat 1,000 milligrams of a mixed fish oil capsule that includes some omega-3s daily. *Vitamin A.* Cats should get enough vitamin A from raw liver if they eat it twice a month as advised above. But a cat who does not eat raw liver should receive a vitamin A supplement. Give one 10,000 IU gel cap twice a week. Cats must have preformed vitamin A instead of beta-carotene, because unlike dogs, they are not able to make vitamin A from its precursor, whether found in supplements or vegetables.

For unwell or ill dogs or cats. If a pet is unwell or ill, other specific supplements may be appropriate. For example, a pet with dysbiotic stress may benefit from added probiotics and enzymes; an allergic animal from added omega-3 oils. But these are therapeutic uses of nutraceuticals and should ideally be addressed in a larger context with the input of a holistic veterinarian.

For pets still on processed foods. If you haven't yet made the shift to an unprocessed diet, your pet should be on the purest, simplest, most industrial chemical-free processed food available and will benefit from an all-purpose natural vitamin and mineral supplement that includes a range of nutrients appropriate to her species.

WHEN CHANGING FROM PROCESSED TO UNPROCESSED FOODS

Some animals switch eagerly to an unprocessed diet and experience little digestive disruption. But some who have eaten processed food all their lives—especially kibble—may not recognize raw meat as food, and others may have looser stools while they adjust. To help these animals make the transition, mix a little of their new diet with their old processed brand at each feeding. Gradually shift the ratio toward totally unprocessed ingredients. Animals whose digestive capacity at first finds unprocessed foods challenging may benefit from probiotics and enzymes added for a while; as their digestion settles down, try backing off the supplements to see if they can handle the raw diet without them.

Be prepared for your animal's stool to change when she moves from a processed to an unprocessed diet. Pets on processed diets tend to have bulky stools, but the stools of those on unprocessed diets are smaller, drier, and lack odor. However, persistent loose stool may be a sign that your pet has dysbiotic stress or a sensitivity to one or more of the items you are feeding her, or both. Either way, these are signs that your pet's living terrain would benefit from holistic support. You may be able to figure out whether she is sensitive to particular foodstuffs by removing one kind of food at a time from her diet and observing for a couple of days to see whether the symptom disappears; if not, then reintroduce that item and remove another, and so on, until you find out which items provoke her to react, and then stop using them. If you're fortunate to have access to bioenergetic assessment, as described in Chapter 6, you could ask your vet to arrange for it as you'll find it faster and easier to discover which foods your pet is sensitive to.

These dietary guidelines were originally inspired by the work of pioneering animal nutrition experts Dr. Ian Billinghurst, Juliette de Baïracli Levy, Richard H. Pitcairn, DVM, PhD, and Susan Hubble Pitcairn. (See Selected Bibliography.) However, just as knowledge about unprocessed diets for dogs and cats continues to evolve, so my clinic's guidelines have evolved from the recommendations of these early advocates. We will no doubt continue to refine our diet protocol over time; check my website at www.newholisticway.com for any significant adjustments we may make to it.

Selected Bibliography

From the great amount of material available, this is but a small sampling of books, articles, and websites that support and promote the approach offered in this book. Visit www.newholisticway.com to see more.

The Stress-Health Connection

Selye, Hans. *Stress Without Distress.* Toronto: McClelland and Stewart Limited, 1974.

Servan-Schreiber, David. *Anti-Cancer: A New Way of Life.* New York: Viking Press, 2008.

Relating to Your Pet

Grandin, Temple and Catherine Johnson. *Animals Make Us Human: Creating the Best Life for Animals.* Orlando: Houghton Mifflin Harcourt, 2009.

Grandin, Temple and Catherine Johnson. *Animals in Translation: Using the Mysteries of Autism to Decode Animal Behavior.* Orlando: Houghton, Mifflin, Harcourt, 2008.

Miller, Pat. *Play with Your Dog.* Wenatchee, Washington: Dogwise Publishing, 2008.

Jay, Silvia. *Dump Dog.* Dogsense Communications, 2007. Available through the author's website at www.voice4dogs.com.

Diet and Food Concerns

Billinghurst, Ian. *Give Your Dog a Bone.* Romford, Essex: Crosskeys Books, 1993.

Kerns, Nancy ed. *The Whole Dog Journal.* Published monthly by the Belvoir Media Group, Palm Coast, Florida. Information:

www.whole-dog-journal.com/. Subscriptions available through www.whole-dog-journal.com/cs.

Levy, Juliette de Baïracli. *The Complete Herbal Handbook for the Dog and Cat.* 6th ed. Reprinted and Corrected. London: Faber and Faber, 1992.

Nestle, Marion. *Pet Food Politics: The Chihuahua in the Coal Mine.* Berkeley: University of California Press, 2008.

Toxins, Pollutants, and Drug Side-Effects

The Environmental Working Group website posts reports that provide extensive discussion of research on environmental pollutants and toxins that affects cats and dogs; see www.ewg.org/reports/pets.

The U.S. Food and Drug Administration Center for Veterinary Medicine posts reports on adverse drug reactions; see www.fda.gov/cvm/ade_cum.htm.

The Veterinary Drugs Directorate (VDD) on Health Canada's website posts information on adverse reactions to veterinary drugs; see www.hc-sc.gc.ca/dhp-mps/vet/advers-react-neg/index-eng.php.

Weinstein, Susan. "Why Vinyl Stinks: If That Vinyl Toy Smells Bad, Chances Are It Contains Toxic Chemicals." *The Whole Dog Journal* 11, no. 4 (April 2008), 12–17.

Winter, Ruth. *A Consumer's Dictionary of Cosmetic Ingredients: Complete Information about the Harmful and Desirable Ingredients Found in Cosmetics and Cosmeceuticals.* New York: Three Rivers Press, 2005.

Immunization

Dodds, W. Jean. "Changing Vaccine Protocols," www.doglogic.com/vaccination.htm (accessed December 17, 2008).

The Rabies Challenge Fund website posts information on rabies vaccination at www.rabieschallengefund.org.

Rodier, Lisa. "Vaccination 101: A Vaccine Researcher Discusses Which Shot He'd Recommend for Your Dog and Which He'd Recommend Avoiding." *The Whole Dog Journal* 11, no. 8 (August 2008), 14–17.

Schultz, Ronald D, R. B. Ford , J. Olsen, and F. Scott. "Titer Testing and Vaccination: A New Look at Traditional Practices." *Veterinary Medicine* 97 (2002), 1–13.

Therapies

Fox, Michael W. *The Healing Touch for Cats: The Proven Massage Program.* Revised edition. New York: Newmarket Press, 2004.

Fox, Michael W. *The Healing Touch for Dogs: The Proven Massage Program for Dogs.* Revised edition. New York: Newmarket Press, 2004.

Trivieri, Larry Jr., and John W. Anderson, eds. *Alternative Medicine: The Definitive Guide.* 2nd ed. Celestial Arts, 2002.

Weinstein, Susan. "Defeating Disease Differently: How Well-informed Owners Pulled Their Dog Through Distemper." *The Whole Dog Journal* 8, no. 11 (November 2005), 12–16.

Selected Resources

Veterinary Holistic Health Care Professional Associations in North America

The Academy of Veterinary Homeopathy
P.O. Box 9280
Wilmington, DE 19809
Phone and Fax: 866-652-1590
www.theavh.org

The American Academy of Veterinary Acupuncture
P.O. Box 1058
Glastonbury, CT 06033
Phone: 860-632-9911; Fax: 860-659-8772
www.aava.org

The American Holistic Veterinary Medical Association
2218 Old Emmorton Road
Bel Air, MD 21015
Phone: 410-569-0795; Fax: 410-569-2346
office@ahvma.org
www.ahvma.org

The American Veterinary Chiropractic Association
442154 E. 140 Road
Bluejacket, OK 74333
Phone: 918-784-2231; Fax: 918-784-2675
www.animalchiropractic.org
www.avcadoctors.com

Veterinary Botanical Medicine Association
6410 Highway 92
Acworth, GA 30102
office@vbma.org
www.vbma.org

Associations in Australia

Australian Association of Holistic Veterinarians
Phone: 02 9431 5000
www.ava.com.au
members@ava.com.au

The Australian Veterinary Acupuncture Group
www.acuvet.com.au

Australian Veterinary Chiropractic Association
P.O. Box 2357
Werribee, VIC 3030
Phone and Fax: 03 9974 1118
www.avca.com.au

Associations in New Zealand

New Zealand Holistic Animal Therapists Association
P.O. Box 186
Whangaparaoa, North Auckland
www.nzhata.org.nz
info@nzhata.org.nz

Associations in the United Kingdom

British Association of Holistic Nutrition and Medicine
Phone: 0845 4651056
www.bahnm.org.uk
secretary@bahnm.org.uk

The British Association of Homeopathic Veterinary Surgeons
c/o Stuart Marston, Secretary-Treasurer
103 Golf Drive
Nuneaton, Warks CV11 6ND
Phone: +44 (0) 7768 322075
www.bahvs.com
sec@bahvs.com

Associations in South Africa

Complementary Vets Organization
Contact: Dr. Jane M. Fraser
Phone: 031 261 4847
fraserjm@mweb.co.za

South African Veterinary Acupuncture Society
Contact information is available through the International Veterinary
Acupuncture Directory at
www.komvet.at//ivadkom/vapsocs.htm

International Associations

The International Veterinary Acupuncture Society
1730 South College Avenue, Suite 301
Fort Collins, CO 80525
Phone: 970-266-0666; Fax: 970-266-0777
www.ivas.org
office@ivas.org

Dr. Paul McCutcheon's Acknowledgments

I want to thank Cindy Kneebone, DVM, my long-term colleague, for selflessly contributing to many facets of this book. The power of your intellect shines daily in our clinic, and your energy for coming up with new ways to diagnose and care for our patients appears endless. Thanks, too, to Sonja Rosic-Banjanin, DVM, my newest colleague, for your valuable input. I am grateful, as well, for the contribution to my practice of Cherri Campbell Dittom, who specializes in auricular medicine. I have been blessed to have a wonderfully supportive clinic staff and on behalf of myself and our patients, I applaud you and all your efforts.

I thank my wife, Jean, for putting up with my preoccupation with this project and enduring my many hours on the phone.

Over so many years, I have been influenced by numerous colleagues, lecturers, and teachers. Thank you all for contributing to my development. I especially acknowledge my many colleagues in the American Holistic Veterinary Medical Association who have helped to support and shape my journey as a holistic veterinarian.

Thanks to my wonderful clients and your fantastic pets for allowing me to be part of your lives.

And to Susan—your persistence, integrity, enthusiasm, and expertise never diminished over a very long journey, and your ability to take my often abstract, poorly expressed ideas and transfer them into logical, palatable, meaningful prose has been exemplary. Thank you for being you.

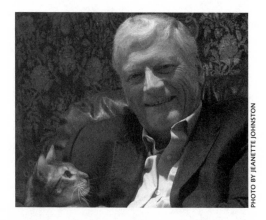

PHOTO BY JEANETTE JOHNSTON

About the Author

PAUL MCCUTCHEON, DVM

Not long after graduating from the Ontario Veterinary College in 1962, Paul McCutcheon had an experience that would transform his career. The cocker spaniel whose ear he was examining had an ear infection. He had been taught that bacteria cause infections. But he had also been taught that healthy animals' ears normally house bacteria. Then why, he wondered, would only one ear be infected? If invasive organisms alone do not cause infections, then treating those organisms with antibiotics alone will not cure the underlying problem. These questions launched his journey toward looking at every individual holistically to discover the stress factors behind all illness.

Intrigued by the ideas of Hans Selye, the internationally renowned medical researcher who illuminated the role of stress in human health, Dr. McCutcheon began to develop a new way of thinking about pet care that focused on stress as the cause of unwellness and illness in cats and dogs. He became the sole veterinarian to speak at the Second International Symposium on Stress Management, in the company of Hans Selye and a number of Nobel Prize winners. He has been a Director of the American Holistic Veterinary Medical Association and named Veterinarian of the Year by his provincial and Canadian professional associations. He has contributed to countless magazines and veterinary journals and hosted his own television and radio shows on pet care. *The New Holistic Way for Dogs & Cats* is his first attempt to provide a full account of his way of thinking about pet care.

Today, his East York Animal Clinic serves about 5,000 patients and employs the services of chiropractors, homeopaths, acupuncturists, and other specialists.

Dr. McCutcheon has been an active member of the Rotary Club since 1962, has raised five children, and now enjoys nine grandchildren. He lives northeast of Toronto with his wife, Jean, and their cats.

Susan Weinstein's Acknowledgments

I have many people to thank for encouraging this book along the way. Among them are Theresa Rickerby and Roberta Jamieson for providing information, resources, and promotional tools; Nancy Kerns, Editor-in-Chief of *The Whole Dog Journal* for her confidence in my work; Claire Polster, Laurel Jackson-White, Wendy Sharko, and Rebekah Theodore for suggestions and feedback; Kim Green for her input; and Danielle Forster, Animal Behaviour Coordinator for the Calgary Humane Society, for research on our behalf. I can't say enough about our agent, Kate Epstein of Epstein Literary Agency upon whose tireless commitment, energy, and advice we have relied. Heartfelt thanks to Julie Bennett for loving the book and ensuring that we made it through the door, and to Veronica Randall, our editor at Ten Speed Press, who saw its significance and potential and for caring as much as she does. I also want to express my gratitude to Paul McCutcheon for his brilliance, inspiration, decency, and good faith. One could not hope to collaborate with a finer individual.

I offer a special acknowledgement to Baron, my Bouvier for waking me at dawn every day and turning me into a morning person so that I could write this book.

Finally, I barely have the words to thank Janice Newson for shouldering more than her share of the cooking, cleaning, and dog-walking, for her generous and clear editorial assistance, for providing me with shelter while I wrote, and for always helping me to find my way through. Her unending support has made this book possible.

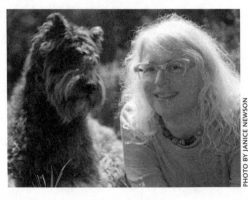

PHOTO BY JANICE NEWSON

About the Author

SUSAN WEINSTEIN

Susan Weinstein has been involved with the welfare of animals since she was twelve. Even before that, she wanted to be a writer. Both of these life-long passions brought her to this collaborative project with Paul McCutcheon, DVM.

Susan's relationship with Dr. McCutcheon began in 1988 when she brought her ailing Bouvier des Flandres dog, Otis, to him for care. She continued on as a client, and in 2004 Susan and Dr. McCutcheon began to plan a book that would be based on his health care philosophy. Their work together culminates in this book.

Susan has a degree in sociology and multidisciplinary studies from York University in Toronto, and writes about issues such as health care, animals, the environment, and democratic education. Along with her writing skill, Susan brings to this project a deep understanding of the environmental, social, and emotional contexts in which humans and their animal friends live together. She gained experience presenting complex ideas about health and encouraging people toward better health care choices through her role in public education about midwifery, and since then through her long-term research on, and use of, holistic health care for herself and her dogs and cats. Her articles on pet care have appeared in *The Whole Dog Journal* and other publications.

Susan lives with her human and animal family in a log house in Eastern Ontario.

Index